the ALZHEIMER'S *health care* HANDBOOK

D0200171

How to Get the Best
Medical Care
for Your Relative with
Alzheimer's Disease,
in and out of the Hospital

MARY S. MITTELMAN, DR.PH & CYNTHIA EPSTEIN, ACSW

MARLOWE & COMPANY
NEW YORK

THE ALZHEIMER'S HEALTH CARE HANDBOOK:
How to Get the Best Medical Care for your Relative with Alzheimer's Disease, in and out of the Hospital

Copyright © 2002, 2003 by Mary S. Mittelman, Dr.PH

Published by
Marlowe & Company
An Imprint of Avalon Publishing Group Incorporated
161 William Street, 16th Floor
New York, NY 10038

Library of Congress Cataloging-in-Publication Data is available.

ISBN 1-56924-445-6

9   8   7   6   5   4   3   2

Printed in the United States of America
Distributed by Publishers Group West

This book is dedicated to the family members, friends, and health care professionals who strive to maintain the health, dignity, and well-being of people with Alzheimer's disease.

This work was funded by grants from the Grotta Foundation, the FJC Foundation, and by the NYU Alzheimer's Disease Center, which is supported by grant P30-AG08051 from the National Institute on Aging.

◆　◆　◆

The Grotta Foundation was created in 1993, charged with the mission of expanding and enhancing services to the elderly of New Jersey and to their families. In the intervening years the Foundation has developed three areas of priority funding. These include: national state and local policy, planning and service innovations that assist family caregivers of the elderly, congregation-based programs for older adults, and technical assistance toward capacity building, coupled with a community small grants program of aging service organizations in Essex, Morris, and Union Counties.

◆　◆　◆

FJC is a foundation of donor advised funds that was founded six years ago by a group of philanthropists to encourage individual philanthropy, maximize charitable resources, and establish innovative programs. FJC has developed the Grant Assistance Program, which enables qualified foreign charities, domestic organizations that have not yet achieved public charity status, and qualified individual artists and writers to receive grants. FJC has also developed the Agency Loan Fund, which assists charities in situations where grant funds are not available. To date, more than 400 donors have established charitable funds at FJC.

◆　◆　◆

The NYU Silberstein Aging and Dementia Research Center, located in New York City, is dedicated to advancing knowledge and understanding of brain aging and Alzheimer's disease and to developing better treatments and care strategies to enhance the well-being of patients and their caregivers. Its programs include the highest quality diagnostic cognitive evaluations and sensitive psychological support, education, and referrals for patients and their family members. Center staff members are experts in the fields of caregiver research and support, clinical trials, neuropsychology, neuroimaging, and psychiatry. More information about the center can be found on their Web site: http://aging.med.nyu.edu/adrc.

CONTENTS

INTRODUCTION   xi

PART ONE
Routine Health Care

1. **How Does Alzheimer's Disease Affect an Individual's Health Care?**   3

   What Is Alzheimer's disease?   3

   What are the stages of Alzheimer's disease?   5

   Are there medical problems caused by Alzheimer's disease?   9

   How does the stage of dementia affect your role As a caregiver?   11

2. **Obtaining Good Health Care for a Person with Alzheimer's Disease.**   13

   Why is it important for people with Alzheimer's disease to get
   regular medical care?   14

   What should you look for in a doctor for a person with
   Alzheimer's disease?   15

   What happens when your family member needs to see
   a specialist?   19

   Why should a patient with Alzheimer's disease get regular
   dental care?   19

   When do you have to restrict the patient's behavior for
   health reasons?   20

3. **The Visit to the Doctor**   22

   How should you prepare for a visit to the doctor?   23

   What can you do to make it easier to take your relative to
   the doctor?   24

   What should you do when you get to the doctor's office?   25

   What should you tell the doctor?   25

   What is your role when your relative is being examined?   26

   What should you do if your relative will not cooperate?   26

4. **Medication and Alzheimer's Disease**   29
   Do you understand the prescription?   30
   What is the role of the pharmacist in medical care?   30
   How can you help your family member take medicine and
      follow a treatment plan?   31
   Are there special medications for Alzheimer's disease?   34

5. **Mental Health Care for a Person with Alzheimer's Disease**   38
   How can you help your family member maintain emotional
      well-being?   39
   Should you tell your family member that he or she has
      Alzheimer's disease?   41
   Should others be told your relative has Alzheimer's disease?   42
   Are there things you should not tell your relative?   43
   What kinds of activities can improve the emotional well-being
      of people with Alzheimer's disease?   44
   Is there treatment for people with Alzheimer's disease who
      are depressed?   45
   What can you do about your relative's disturbing behavior?   46
   Where can you go for help?   47

6. **Who Will Make Medical Decisions for a Person with Alzheimer's Disease?**   48
   Can people with Alzheimer's disease make medical
      decisions for themselves?   49
   Should you include your family member in making
      medical decisions?   49
   What are advance directives?   51
   Who can help you make medical decisions for your relative?   53

PART TWO:

Preparing for a Hospitalization

7. **The Profile of the Person with Memory Impairment**   57
   What is the *Profile of the Person with Memory Impairment?*   58
   Who should use the *Profile of the Person with Memory Impairment?*   59
   How can the *Profile of the Person with Memory Impairment*
      be used?   59

8. **Planning Before the Crisis Comes**   61
   What is a crisis kit?   62
   Who will go to the hospital with your family member if
      you are not available?   63
   Who will stay with your relative in the hospital?   64
   What should you ask your relative's doctor in advance?   65
   What should you know about the hospital?   66

What will the insurance company require?   67
What if you are caring for more than one disabled person?   67
What else can you plan in advance?   68

9. **What to Do in an Emergency**   69

Is this an emergency?   69
What if you are not there when an emergency occurs?   71
How should your family member get to the hospital?   72
What should you do while waiting for the ambulance?   72
What should you do when the ambulance arrives?   73
What hospital will the ambulance go to?   74
What will happen in the ambulance? 74

10. **In the Emergency Room**   75

Why do people go to the emergency room?   75
What will happen in the emergency room?   76
What is your role in the emergency room?   78
Will your family member be admitted to the hospital?   80
Will you need extra support in the emergency room or
    afterwards?   81

11. **What to Do When Hospitalization is Recommended**   83

Is there an alternative to hospitalization?   84
Should you follow the doctor's recommendations?   85
What should you ask the doctor before your relative goes
    to the hospital?   86
How can you prepare your relative for a hospital stay?   87
How can you prepare yourself for the hospitalization?   88

PART THREE
In the Hospital

12. **The Effect of Hospitalization on a Person with Alzheimer's Disease**   91

Why is being in the hospital especially difficult for people with
    Alzheimer's disease?   92
What effect does the stage of dementia have on a person's
    behavior in the hospital?   93
What special needs do people with Alzheimer's disease have
    when they are in the hospital?   95

13. **An Introduction to Your Role As a Caregiver in the Hospital**   96

Why should you tell the hospital staff that your relative
    has dementia?   97
What can you do for your hospitalized relative?   98
Can you do it all alone?   100

14. **Taking Care of Yourself**   101

How can you pace yourself?   101

What can you do to make yourself more comfortable in
the hospital?   102

What kinds of social support can you look for in the
hospital?   103

What about all those feelings?   104

15. **Decisions**   106

Who makes decisions for a person with Alzheimer's
disease?   107

What kinds of decisions can you expect to make?   108

Who can help you make decisions?   110

Should you approve a particular procedure?   111

Should you ask for a second opinion?   112

16. **Supervising Your Family Member in the Hospital**   114

What kind of special help does your family member need? 115

How much supervision does your family member need?   117

How can you arrange for enough help in the hospital?   117

How do you go about hiring help?   118

17. **Working with the Hospital Staff**   121

What is the best way to build a relationship with the hospital
staff?   122

What will the hospital staff expect from you?   122

How can you communicate effectively with the hospital
staff?   123

How can you help the hospital staff understand and care for
your family member?   124

Who can help if you have a problem?   125

18. **How to Make Your Relative More Comfortable in the Hospital Room** 128

How can you arrange the hospital room for a person with
Alzheimer's disease?   129

What are some strategies for managing common behavior
problems?   130

What can you do if your relative becomes agitated?   131

What if your relative is verbally or physically aggressive?   132

What can you do if your relative has problems with
other patients in the room?   134

19. **What is Your Role in the Treatment Process?**   136

How can you help the hospital staff communicate with
your family member?   137

How can you help your family member cooperate with
      medical care in the hospital?   138
What do you need to know about problems people with
      dementia have with medication?   140
What should you do if your relative must stay in bed?   142

20. Preparing for Discharge from the Hospital   143

What is a discharge plan and how is it developed?   144
What does a discharge plan include?   144
Where will your relative go after the hospital stay?   146

PART FOUR

After the Hospital

21. When Your Relative Is Discharged Home   151

How can you prepare the home for your relative's return?   152
What kinds of services will your relative get at home?   154
What if your relative needs complicated medical equipment or
      treatment after discharge?   157
What if additional home care is needed?   157
What if it becomes too difficult to care for your relative at
      home?   159

22. If Your Relative Cannot Go Directly Home   160

Where can a person get short-term care after a hospital stay?   161
What if nursing home placement is recommended?   162
What other living arrangements are available for a person with
      Alzheimer's disease?   163
What should you look for in a facility?   164
How can you and your relative adjust to the change in living
      arrangements?   165

23. The Death of a Person with Alzheimer's Disease   167

What will you do when your relative's death is near?   168
How can you follow your relative's advance directives?   168
What is palliative care?   169
What is hospice care?   169
Should your relative receive palliative care?   170
What should you do when your relative dies?   170
Should an autopsy of your relative's brain be performed?   171
And now, you . . . ?   172

APPENDIX   174
    Definition of terms commonly used on prescriptions   174
    Description of hospital and support personnel   175
    Profile of a Person with Memory Impairment   178

GUIDE TO RESOURCES   184
ACKNOWLEDGMENTS   191
INDEX   193

INTRODUCTION

It is easy enough to say that staying healthy is important, but trying to achieve this goal for a family member suffering from Alzheimer's disease can be an enormous challenge. Some of the many problems that occur are caused by the symptoms of the illness, which worsen over time. Others result from the fact that the health care system is not geared to meet the special needs of a person with Alzheimer's or other dementia. That is why we have written this guide—to help you, the family caregiver, overcome some of these problems. We believe that if you know what to expect, make the necessary plans, and get adequate support, you will be able to insure the best medical care for a person with Alzheimer's disease— a crucial part of caregiving.

The guide—complete with facts, tips, and strategies—will give you the information you need to provide routine health care, plan for a hospitalization, help your relative and the hospital staff to communicate during a hospitalization, and finally to make aftercare and end-of-life decisions. You are, of course, invited to read it from beginning to end; but it is also designed so that you can turn directly to those sections that you may need at the moment. It also shows you how to use two caregiving innovations— the *Profile of a Person with Memory Impairment* and the Crisis Kit—that can reduce some of the stresses of caregiving. With that in mind, be sure not to skip the chapter on taking care of yourself. It is every bit as important as those dealing with the care of your family member.

The guide is divided into four parts. In Part One, we discuss the routine health care of a person with Alzheimer's disease. Ideally the care you provide will enable your family member to remain healthy. But even with the best of care, people get sick and need to go to the hospital. Part Two describes the steps you can take in advance so that a hospitalization will take the least toll on you and your family member. Whether it is the result of a crisis or has been planned in advance, being in a hospital can be extremely trying for people with AD and their family caregivers. Part Three focuses on how to work within the hospital environment to assure the best care for a person with AD. Finally, in Part Four, we discuss what happens when your family member leaves the hospital, either to return home or enter a care facility. It is intended to help you adjust to both possibilities and, when the inevitable happens, to know your options for end-of-life care and, ultimately, the end of your caregiving. At the back of the book, you will find a glossary of terms commonly used in prescriptions, a list of hospital personnel explaining the role each in patient care, and a number of resources for further information, assistance, and support.

Caring for a person with AD can touch your heart and often break it. Be prepared to have mixed and contradictory feelings, especially when your family member is sick and you are more worried and tired than usual. You may find yourself feeling full of love for your family member one minute, and full of anger and frustration a few minutes later. All these reactions are understandable and normal.

Our hope is that this book will help you overcome the many obstacles that caregivers face as they try to maintain the physical and emotional health of a person with Alzheimer's disease.

PART ONE

◆   ◆   ◆

Routine Health Care

· 1 ·

How Does Alzheimer's Disease Affect an Individual's Health Care?

Some older people experience serious changes in memory, thinking, and behavior that are significant enough to get in the way of the everyday things they do. Many words—such as *senility*, *second childhood*, and *hardening of the arteries*—have been used to describe these changes. They are, however, not just the result of normal aging, but signs of an illness that health professionals commonly call *dementia*. The most common cause of dementia in the elderly is Alzheimer's disease.

> IN THIS CHAPTER
>
> What Is Alzheimer's Disease?
>
> What Are the Stages of Alzheimer's Disease?
>
> Are There Medical Problems Caused by Alzheimer's Disease?
>
> How Does the Stage of Dementia Affect Your Role As a Caregiver?

WHAT IS ALZHEIMER'S DISEASE?

Alzheimer's disease is a neurological illness that prevents the brain from functioning effectively. The earliest symptoms are memory problems.

Later on there are problems with concentration, attention span, speech, mood, and behavior. Eventually the ability to control the body is lost.

The cause of Alzheimer's disease (which is often abbreviated as AD) is still unknown. It is not contagious and, in most cases, not hereditary.

There are other illnesses that cause dementia in the elderly. Many of their symptoms are similar to those of AD, although their course and treatment may be different. We will use the terms *Alzheimer's disease*, *AD*, and *dementia* interchangeably in this book.

AD is a progressive disease, which means it gets worse over time. Early in the course of the illness it may be difficult to recognize that a person has Alzheimer's. This is because the memory loss is usually mild and appears to get better and worse at various times and in different circumstances. As the symptoms worsen, however, it eventually becomes clear that something is definitely wrong.

If you are unsure whether your relative has AD, a comprehensive evaluation of his or her physical and cognitive status can clarify the situation. The sooner you find out why your relative is having these symptoms, the sooner you both can get appropriate information and help.

◆　◆　◆

Janet is in her seventies. She lives with her husband in the same town as her widowed sister, Margaret, who is six years older than she. About three months ago, Margaret started calling Janet several times a day, asking about appointments she had made with doctors or friends.

"She asks me for the directions over and over again, but when I offer to go with her or to help in any way, she just acts offended and says that she is perfectly fine."

Janet admits she does not always remember things herself, but the problems Margaret is having seem different. "When I ask her if she is eating properly, she insists that she is and just gets huffy with me. But the last time I was at her house, most of the food in the refrigerator was spoiled. Margaret has always been an excellent housekeeper, but her bed wasn't made, and the vacuum cleaner was in the middle of the living room."

Janet is worried about Margaret, especially since she lives alone, but is not sure what is causing her sister to behave this way, and hopes she will be able to convince her to see a doctor.

◆　◆　◆

DEFINITIONS

We will try not to use technical medical terms in this book, but it may be helpful for you to understand some of the words health care professionals may use when talking about your relative with AD. Here are some words you should know:

Acute: Sudden, severe, and temporary; the opposite of chronic.

Behavioral: Related to the way people act.

Chronic: Lasting a long time; usually incurable, though not necessarily fatal.

Cognitive: Related to mental processes; the way people think, perceive, reason, remember, and judge things; how the mind works.

Delirium: A sudden, but temporary, change in the way a person thinks and behaves. Its many causes include physical illness (especially if the person has a fever), pain, reactions to drugs, head injury, and alcohol abuse.

Dementia: Impaired ability to think and remember that interferes with normal activity. Unlike delirium, dementia is usually permanent and, in the case of Alzheimer's disease, will get progressively worse.

Neurological: Related to the nervous system; including the brain, spinal cord, and network of nerves throughout the body.

Progressive: A disease or condition that worsens over time in contrast to one that is temporary, unchanging, or reversible.

Symptom: A noticeable sign of a disease or abnormal condition.

WHAT ARE THE STAGES OF ALZHEIMER'S DISEASE?

For convenience, we talk about Alzheimer's disease as having stages, and of people progressing from stage to stage. In this book, we will refer to people as being in the *mild, moderate, moderately severe,* or *very severe* stages of AD.

The symptoms of AD appear gradually, over the course of many years, because of increasing damage to nerve cells and connections in the brain.

Knowing the order in which the symptoms usually occur and what is typical of each stage will help you plan for the care of your relative and prepare yourself for what is likely to happen next. Whenever you notice a new symptom or behavior that is not typical of the stage he or she is in, you should tell the doctor, since it may not be related to AD. For example, incontinence tends to occur at the end of the moderate stage. If your relative is in the mild stage and becomes incontinent, the problem is probably being caused by another condition, one that should be investigated and, if possible, treated.

But the description of the stages of dementia is only a guideline. The disease does not develop in each person in exactly the same way. Your family member may have symptoms of more than one stage at the same time, or never develop some symptoms at all.

MILD DEMENTIA

The earliest stage of Alzheimer's disease can last for many years. People in this stage:

- Experience memory problems.
- Forget things shortly after they happen.
- Have trouble concentrating.
- May not be able to handle finances as well as before.
- May not be able to shop as well as before.
- May not be able to plan social events.
- May express depressed thoughts and feelings.

People in the mild stage of AD may be easily frustrated when they cannot solve problems or figure out what to do next. Small changes in their routine or environment may throw them off balance. If they have trouble with language, for instance, it will be hard for them to understand what is being said or express their needs. Sometimes they will get irritable, worried, and agitated as a result of their limitations. Some will deny that they are having any problems at all, but stay away from situations they find too difficult to handle in order to maintain the illusion that everything is normal.

People in this stage may describe events and experiences in such a realistic way that a listener would never guess that many parts of the story are untrue. They are not doing this to deceive, but because it is too painful to admit even to themselves that they cannot remember what actually happened.

Still, many people in the mild stage can manage fairly well on their own. They continue to live alone, remain interested, and participate in many of their usual activities.

MODERATE DEMENTIA

People in this stage may:

- Still dress, bathe, eat, and use the toilet without help.
- Get lost if they leave the house on their own.
- Need help choosing the correct clothing.
- Get anxious about upcoming events.
- Be afraid of being left alone.
- Have trouble following directions.
- Experience delusions and hallucinations.
- Blame others for difficulties they experience in finding or doing things.

DEFINITIONS

Delusion: A false belief that a person holds onto in spite of good evidence that it is not correct.

Hallucination: An experience of seeing, hearing, feeling, or smelling something that is not there.

Paranoia: Suspiciousness that certain situations or people may be harmful. These beliefs may lead to falsely accusing someone of stealing or being unfaithful.

People in the moderate stage cannot get along without the help of another person. They may, however, sometimes become irritable and angry with the people who care for them, while still acting like their old selves with strangers.

MODERATELY SEVERE DEMENTIA

People with moderately severe dementia become much more dependent. In this stage, they may:

- Not dress appropriately or bathe correctly without help.
- Not finish things they have started.
- Wander or pace.
- Have difficulty communicating (finding words, sticking to the subject, talking sensibly).
- Behave or speak aggressively.
- Have hallucinations or delusions.
- Be paranoid.
- Be reluctant to bathe and unable to attend to other aspects of hygiene.
- Curse or make inappropriate sexual references or gestures.
- Begin to lose control of bowel and bladder functions, having frequent accidents.

Changes in personality and emotional reactions become very obvious in the moderately severe stage. You may find yourself thinking or saying, "He just doesn't seem like himself anymore," or "That's so unlike her." Irritability and anxiety are common as confusion increases. People in this stage have trouble understanding, following directions from, and cooperating with those taking care of them. You will therefore need to be responsible for making most decisions and insuring the physical safety and cleanliness of your relative when he or she gets to this stage.

VERY SEVERE DEMENTIA

People at this stage lose the ability to:

- Speak.
- Walk.
- Swallow (and forget to chew).
- Smile.
- Hold up their heads.

When people with AD reach the very severe stage, they require complete physical care and depend on others for help all the time. As this stage progresses, they eventually lose all ability to function.

ARE THERE MEDICAL PROBLEMS CAUSED BY ALZHEIMER'S DISEASE?

Because AD is almost always a disease of old age, people suffering from it tend to have other age-related health problems as well. But the disease itself—the progressive neurological damage—can cause specific medical problems or make existing ones worse. Those more likely to occur in people with AD than in other elderly people include delirium and eating disorders, which can appear at any stage of AD; and incontinence and immobility, which are generally found only in the more severe stages.

DELIRIUM: At all stages of the disease, people with dementia are more likely to develop delirium when they are physically ill, have a bad reaction to medication or anesthesia, or are under severe physical or emotional stress.

Delirium is a state of confusion that affects thought, speech, movement, and perception. People who are delirious may not know where they are or remember what you tell them. They may be unusually restless and upset, and may sometimes think they see things that are not there.

Delirium looks a lot like severe dementia. Unlike dementia, however, delirium comes on suddenly and goes away when whatever has caused it is corrected. The person who has suffered an attack may be in physical danger if left alone and unsupervised. When it is over, he or she will have no memory of it, but it can be extremely frightening to a caregiver. (In Chapter 18, we will offer advice on how to handle delirium and other dangerous behavior.)

EATING DISORDERS: Although they may no longer be able to shop or prepare their own food, most people in the mild stage of AD can still make good food choices; even those in the moderate stage may continue to feed themselves. (In Chapter 2, we will talk more about how to help your relative maintain a healthy life style.)

In the moderately severe stage, however, people may forget that they have eaten and need to be distracted from wanting the meal they have just had. Others lose interest in eating and need to be coaxed.

People in the very severe stage can no longer feed themselves. They may need to eat pureed food and be reminded to swallow. The inability to swallow associated with this last stage may cause life-threatening malnutrition and dehydration. When a person can no longer eat enough to maintain adequate nutrition, caregivers will have to decide whether or not to have a feeding tube inserted. The decision to use invasive measures such as this is a very difficult one for a family caregiver to make. Hopefully, your relative will have prepared *advance directives* (see Chapter 6) so that the decision will have been made for you.

INCONTINENCE: People in the moderate to moderately severe stages gradually become incontinent. Many family caregivers fear that they will not be able to handle this difficult and embarrassing situation. Most, however, are able to overcome their initial negative reaction.

MOVEMENT PROBLEMS: There are no obvious physical signs of AD in the early stages of the disease. As it progresses, some people begin to have poor balance, show signs of muscle rigidity, and are more likely to fall and possibly break a bone. If muscles are not exercised, painful contractures—tightening of the muscles that cause irreversible deformities of the joints—make it impossible for the person to move comfortably or at all. People in the very severe stage, who may no longer be able to get out of bed on their own, are also vulnerable to pressure (or bed) sores and pneumonia unless they are moved and their muscles regularly exercised.

The changes that often come in the later stages can be delayed or, in some cases, even prevented by a good exercise program early on. Regular exercise (walking, stretching, even swimming, and lifting light weights, if appropriate) should be part of routine preventive health care and continue for as long as possible. Such an exercise program is not only good insurance against movement problems, but can also improve mood, give structure to the day, and provide increased opportunities for companionship.

HOW DOES THE STAGE OF DEMENTIA AFFECT YOUR ROLE AS A CAREGIVER?

The stage of dementia will affect a person's ability to care for him or herself and to cooperate when others provide care. It will also affect the way he or she is perceived by doctors and other health care professionals.

In the mild stage, your role will mainly be to help your relative remember what needs to be done. For example, you will have to remind him or her about doctors' appointments and when and how to take medications. At this stage of the illness, the dementia may not be immediately obvious. You may have to tell doctors that your relative has memory problems and may not remember to follow instructions.

In the later stages, you will have more responsibility for your family member's medical well-being, like accompanying him or her to the doctor, preparing or giving medications, and generally making more and eventually all the medical decisions. Finally, the day will arrive when constant supervision and hands-on care are needed.

◆   ◆   ◆

Mr. C struggles with the reality of his wife's Alzheimer's. "My wife looks just like she always did. She dresses beautifully, goes to the beauty parlor, and sounds really intelligent. Sometimes I just can't believe she has Alzheimer's. I think that if I don't tell anyone maybe they won't catch on and our life can go on the way it always did."

Increasingly, however, Mr. C knows that there are decisions he cannot leave up to his wife anymore. "She just forgets to do things and then makes all kinds of excuses. Sometimes she even makes up stories that sound so true I would believe them myself if I didn't know better. She told the doctor that she never had any operations, never was in the hospital, and that she doesn't take any medications. I guess she forgot how sick she was just a few years ago."

Mr. C realizes that from now on he will have to go with his wife to medical appointments to be sure the doctor gets the real story and to hear first hand what the doctor has to say.

◆   ◆   ◆

Since Alzheimer's is a progressive disease, your relative will require more and more care as time goes on. You may choose to provide most of the care yourself or arrange for others to do so all or part of the time. This may involve getting help from other family members and friends or hiring someone to assist with caregiving. In the chapters that follow, we will look at the tasks and situations that you will face in providing the best possible health care for a person who is suffering from Alzheimer's.

◆ 2 ◆

Obtaining Good Health Care for a Person with Alzheimer's Disease

People with Alzheimer's disease suffer from the same illnesses and disabilities as other elderly people. Although it is harder to make sure that someone with AD gets routine medical care, such care will pay off in many ways. For one thing, it is always easier and better to prevent medical problems than to treat them. Then again, people with AD cannot be counted on to be entirely responsible for their own medical care, even in the mild stage. They cannot think as well as they used to. This means, for example, that they may not remember which medications to take or how to follow a special diet. In this chapter, we will discuss why it is important to provide good routine medical care for a person with AD and the steps caregivers can take to obtain such care.

IN THIS CHAPTER

Why Is It Important for People with Alzheimer's Disease to Get Regular Medical Care?

What Should You Look for in a Doctor for a Person with Alzheimer's Disease?

What Happens When Your Family Member Needs to See a Specialist?

Why Should a Patient with Alzheimer's Disease Get Regular Dental Care?

When Do You Have to Restrict Your Family Member's Behavior for Health Reasons?

WHY IS IT IMPORTANT FOR PEOPLE WITH ALZHEIMER'S DISEASE TO GET REGULAR MEDICAL CARE?

Regular preventive measures, many of which are partially or fully paid for by Medicare, are as important for people with AD as for anyone else who is elderly. In addition to following a good diet, getting enough exercise, and being involved in meaningful activities, they periodically should have:

- General medical checkups, including blood pressure, cholesterol, EKG, and blood chemistry, and screening for diabetes.
- Dental care, including fitting and maintenance of dentures.
- Eye examinations, including filling new prescriptions for eyeglasses.
- Hearing evaluations, including fitting and maintenance of hearing aids.
- Annual flu and pneumonia vaccinations.
- Appropriate cancer screening, including—
    Mammograms and physical breast examinations.
    Pap smears and gynecological examinations.
    Tests and examinations for cancer of the colon, rectum, and prostate.

Promptly treating any health problems that arise is also extremely important since untreated physical illnesses are particularly serious for people with AD, making them more confused and causing a great deal of avoidable distress. For this reason, you should act quickly and take your family member to the doctor at the first sign of illness.

Even during routine visits, the doctor will be able to identify problems your relative may be unable to tell you about, such as vision or hearing impairment, mouth pain, or ill-fitting dentures. It is not unusual for mild dehydration, severe constipation, urinary tract or other infection, or even a broken bone to be discovered during a routine medical examination. Discomfort from these and other conditions can be responsible for what appears to be difficult behavior. Sometimes when the physical causes are corrected, people with AD are less confused, in better moods, and more able to interact with those around them. When not identified, these same conditions frequently get worse and bring a person with AD to the emergency room.

Finally, be sure that there is a first-aid kit readily available to take care of the minor accidents that happen to everyone. Keep the kit and the patient's other medicines handy. Make sure everyone who spends time with your relative knows where they are, but keep them out of reach of the person with AD, if he or she is too impaired to know how to use them.

◆　　◆　　◆

When Mr. W developed heart disease, his wife took care of him. But as Mr. W declined and Mrs. W started to show signs of Alzheimer's, their son Robert had to get more involved and began to accompany them to their medical appointments.

"They had a lovely internist, who was also a cardiologist, so he treated both of them. But oh what a secretary he had! Dealing with her was enough to induce cardiac arrest. So could the double doors and the two short flights of steps you had to deal with to get into the office. I vowed that I would stick with this doctor as long as my father needed him, but not one day more."

After Mr. W died, Robert began looking for another doctor for his mother, and eventually found one who was kind and respectful, understood dementia, answered telephone calls, and even asked Robert how he was. "Sometimes I think I will burst into tears just from the relief of not having to fight for every little bit of help."

◆　　◆　　◆

WHAT SHOULD YOU LOOK FOR IN A DOCTOR FOR A PERSON WITH ALZHEIMER'S DISEASE?

It is very important for a person with AD to have a regular doctor who understands the medical needs of elderly people and specifically the treatment of this disease. Geriatricians, who are specialists in aging, have the necessary combination of skills and experience, but so do many general or family practitioners.

Whether your family member already has a doctor and you are just beginning to get involved or are looking for a new doctor, you might schedule a private appointment during which the two of you can discuss your relative's needs. That will give you a chance to see how well the doctor's approach and philosophy match your own and how well you can work together. If you do not feel comfortable with your relative's current doctor, it is a good idea to find a new one. Ask other family caregivers whom they use or call your local Alzheimer's Association for a referral.

Look for a doctor who is kind and patient and with whom you and your family member feel comfortable. This is at least as important as an office with the most up-to-date equipment. While only mildly impaired by AD, your relative may want to talk to the doctor about how he or she and the family feel about the illness. The doctor can also help your relative and family discuss, in advance, the many medical care decisions that may need to be made when he or she can no longer express these wishes. A doctor who is gentle, speaks softly, and has a caring manner can develop a good relationship with your relative and also be an enormous source of support for the entire family.

It is essential to know in advance how much the physician is willing to involve you and your relative with AD in medical decisions. Some physicians feel that the autonomy of the patient is so important that they will suggest that your relative make decisions about medical care when you, the caregiver, feel that it is no longer appropriate. Others may begin to ignore the views of their patient sooner than you would. Keep in mind that even people who are very confused about many things still have a right to contribute to the decision-making process. They can communicate their opinion if they are questioned skillfully. It will be worth the effort to find a physician who shares your views.

◆   ◆   ◆

Although he is in the moderate stage of AD, Mr. N continues to use the telephone. In fact, as far as his daughter is concerned, he uses it too much. "My father seems to have entered the moderate stage of AD with a telephone in his hand. I am kind of amazed that he can actually manage to make the calls because he is so confused about so many things."

Once he gets an idea in his head, he can spend an entire day calling his doctors and telling the person who answers the phone that something or other hurts him and he wants to make an appointment. It is almost impossible to divert him from this mission when he is in this mood. Fortunately, his doctors already know he has AD, as do their staffs. Since Mr. N's daughter chose doctors who understand the effects of AD, everyone is very kind when he calls.

Still, his daughter always wonders if something her father cannot explain is actually hurting him. "When I ask him if his head hurts or his stomach or his foot, he always says he doesn't know. Sometimes I take him to his doctor for an exam just to check him out. So far, the doctor has never found anything. I always leave the office promising myself that I won't bring him again for what appears to be no reason. But since you can never be sure and you don't want to ignore a problem, I'll probably end up taking him again the next time he starts complaining."

◆   ◆   ◆

CHOOSING A DOCTOR

The ideal primary care physician for a person with Alzheimer's Disease should:

- Have experience treating patients with dementia.
- Answer and return telephone calls.
- Be willing to spend time talking with you.
- Be able to communicate with your relative.
- Be willing to consult with experts.
- Be willing to coordinate the care provided by specialists.
- Know about new treatments for dementia.
- Be aware of relevant clinical trials.

The doctor should make you feel that it is okay to call if you have questions or need help. A short conversation on the telephone may be enough to put your mind at ease or catch a problem before it gets serious.

A phone call may save you a visit to the doctor's office. Of course, you have to be careful not to overuse the privilege.

HEALTH CARE OUTSIDE A DOCTOR'S OFFICE

Alternative ways to get medical care are provided by:

- Some **adult day care programs**.
- **Nurse practitioners**, who are now available in many communities, offer many of the same services as doctors, and may spend more time with each patient.

If leaving home is too stressful or otherwise impractical:

- Agencies such as the **Visiting Nurse Service,** with a referral from a physician, will send a nurse to examine your family member and inform the doctor about his or her medical condition so the doctor can take the appropriate steps. Depending on the nurse's report, the doctor may decide it is necessary to see your relative after all.
- There are also physicians who make house calls. Phone your local hospital or Alzheimer's Association chapter for a referral.

A doctor's time is limited by the pressure to see many patients, so it is wise to develop other relationships and resources for non-medical information.

- **The Alzheimer's Association** has a wealth of knowledge about the disease in general as well as local and national resources. It is also a source of referrals for many of your needs as a caregiver.
- A **geriatric social worker,** who is affiliated with a community agency or with whom you are able to work privately, can help with issues such as your reactions to caregiving and to the patient's behavior, and developing a support system.
- **Support group**s for family caregivers can be a rich source of information and resources.

WHAT HAPPENS WHEN YOUR FAMILY MEMBER NEEDS TO SEE A SPECIALIST?

There will be times when the primary care physician will recommend that your relative see a specialist. For example, a geriatric psychiatrist (one who specializes in treating the elderly) may be the best person to consult about treatment and management of mood and behavior disturbances in people with AD. A neurologist may be consulted if there is a question about whether a physical change, such as the inability to use a limb, is related to the AD or another illness.

One of the jobs of the primary care physician is to coordinate care. When the doctor says your family member should be seen by a specialist in a hurry, he or she may offer to call for an appointment. If this is not offered, ask. Having the physician call the specialist may help you get an appointment quickly, and allow the physician to explain your relative's condition in detail.

You should tell the specialists at the time appointments are made that your family member has dementia. This may influence how they approach him or her and the treatment they recommend. Specialists who regularly treat patients with dementia will have experience using the most suitable techniques. For example, a patient with AD may not be able to read an eye chart. It will be helpful if the ophthalmologist has an instrument that measures vision automatically without relying on the response of the person being examined.

WHY SHOULD A PATIENT WITH ALZHEIMER'S DISEASE GET REGULAR DENTAL CARE?

Routine dental care—regular cleaning and checkups of tooth and gum health—is important for people with AD. If their teeth or dentures are well maintained, they will have an easier time eating and speaking. They will also be more attractive to the people around them and feel better about themselves.

Still, it can be a challenge to provide dental care for patients with AD. Sometimes they refuse to open their mouths. They may bite down when they should not. They may not be able to tell you when dentures do not fit properly or when they have a toothache. Nevertheless, dental care is essential, so look for a dentist who has experience treating patients with dementia.

When your family member can no longer take care of his or her own teeth, you (or someone else) will need to help. At first you may only have to offer a reminder or provide a toothbrush. Later on in the illness, the brushing or denture cleaning will have to be done by a caregiver. Unless it is done regularly, your relative may refuse to let anyone help with daily dental care or allow someone's hands in his or her mouth. Then dental care will become even more difficult.

WHEN DO YOU HAVE TO RESTRICT THE PATIENT'S BEHAVIOR FOR HEALTH REASONS?

People with AD may have had problems with alcohol abuse or recreational drugs before they became ill. These substances sometimes can cause dementia or make the symptoms worse. If your relative uses alcohol or recreational drugs and is unwilling to stop, it may be wisest to just make sure that they are no longer available. This may mean asking family members, friends, and anyone else who interacts with your relative not to give in to any requests.

If alcohol is a problem, it is best not to drink when your family member is around, or to offer a substitute such as sparkling cider, ginger ale, or nonalcoholic beer during social situations so he or she does not feel left out. If your family member can still go out alone, consider asking personnel in local stores to let you know if he or she has purchased alcohol. The alcohol problem will probably disappear, since people in the later stages of AD generally forget about it.

Smoking is dangerous to everyone's health, but it poses additional hazards for people with AD, who may forget that they have left a cigarette or a match burning and cause a fire. If your relative smokes, make every effort to encourage him or her to quit. Failing that, try to make smoking materials less available, and make sure someone is present when he or she smokes.

Your relative's diet may need to be controlled to avoid excessive weight gain or loss or nutritional deficiencies. Many people with AD need to follow a special diet because of other illnesses such as diabetes or high cholesterol. Those who live alone may stop shopping, not realize when food is spoiled, or be unable to cope in the kitchen as well as they used to. They also may forget that they have just eaten and eat again or forget to eat altogether.

In the early stages of the illness, your relative may be willing to eat at the many senior centers that serve food, or to have services such as Meals on Wheels deliver food to the home. Some families leave a selection of pre-pared food in the freezer. Since people with AD often forget they have food heating on the stove, it may be helpful to get a very simple microwave oven. However, even a microwave is not problem free, since only certain types of containers and utensils can be used safely. When your family member progresses into the moderate stage of the illness, the preparation and serving of food will have to be handled by another person.

It is important to make changes in the environment that will keep your relative out of harm's way. Locking certain cabinets, hiding foods that are not appropriate, and creating distractions with an acceptable activity may prevent accidents from happening to a person with demen-tia who cannot control the effects of the disease on his or her behavior.

As people with AD are less and less able to manage activities of daily life on their own, they will need to have someone look in on them regu-larly and eventually stay with them at least part of the time. Taking care of the health of a person with AD can be as burdensome as it is essential. As the dementia progresses and care becomes more difficult, having a sensitive, trusted, skillful, and accessible primary care physician will greatly reduce your stress, while meeting your relative's health needs. In the chapters that follow, we will look at some of those needs and the ways in which you can assure that they are met.

· 3 ·

The Visit to the Doctor

You know it is important for your family member with Alzheimer's disease to receive good health care, but that does not mean it is easy. Getting to a doctor's office is only the first step. What you and your relative do once you are there and how you both feel about it can make or break an entire day. Even a routine visit to the doctor may cause a person with Alzheimer's disease to feel anxious. A change in the regular schedule and the need to be dressed and out of the house on time can be stressful for both of you, but there are ways of making a medical office visit go more smoothly.

IN THIS CHAPTER

How Should You Prepare for a Visit to the Doctor?

What Can You Do to Make It Easier to Take Your Relative to the Doctor?

What Should You Do When You Get to the Doctor's Office?

What Should You Tell the Doctor?

What Is Your Role When Your Relative Is Being Examined?

What Should You Do If Your Relative Will Not Cooperate?

HOW SHOULD YOU PREPARE FOR A VISIT
TO THE DOCTOR?

The more details that you can take care of in advance, the more able you will be to give your full attention to your family member when you are in the doctor's office. The first step in advance planning is a phone call. You need information from the doctor's office, and the office staff needs information from you.

If this is an initial visit, explain your family member's special needs. Ask for an appointment at a time when the office is less likely to be busy, and waiting times are more likely to be short. With luck, this will also be a time of day when your relative feels most comfortable.

First-time patients are usually asked to fill out a questionnaire with information about insurance, date of birth, medical history, and current medications, among other details. Ask if you can provide this information over the phone or send it in before your visit. If reports or test results from another doctor are needed, make sure they are forwarded in time for the appointment, or bring them along yourself.

In Chapter 7, we describe a form called the *Profile of the Person with Alzheimer's Disease*. It is designed to help you give a complete description of your relative with dementia, including medical status and care needs, to those who do not know him or her. If you have the time before the next doctor's appointment, complete this form and either send or give it to the doctor.

Let the secretary or office manager know in advance that you want to have copies of any laboratory results, such as blood and urine tests, and reports from such procedures as MRI, mammogram, and EKG. Having a copy of your relative's medical records, including all test results, will save time and probably aggravation when you go to a new physician or specialist. A loose leaf binder can help keep them in order.

Discuss the method of payment. Will the doctor expect to be paid immediately, send you the bill, or bill the insurance company directly? May you pay with a credit card?

If you take your relative with AD to a physician on a regular basis, you will know the office procedures, and the physician and office staff will know your relative and understand the special problems dementia creates. The office staff can help by scheduling appointments at convenient times and distracting or comforting your relative if he or she gets upset in the office.

WHAT CAN YOU DO TO MAKE IT EASIER TO TAKE YOUR RELATIVE TO THE DOCTOR?

People in the mild stage of AD may need to be reminded that they have an appointment with the doctor. They may think they can find the doctor's office on their own, but get lost on the way. In later stages, when people cannot go by themselves, they may seem to be uncooperative every step of the way. They may move more slowly than usual and ask the same questions over and over: "Where are we going? Why are we going? Are we there yet?" Or they may simply refuse to leave the house despite the fact that you have waited weeks for an appointment with a specialist. This can be especially frustrating for you. Try to remember that people with AD may not be able to understand why it is so important to go to the doctor. But do not give up!

If your family member is physically ill, the symptoms of AD—anger, suspicion, fear—may be more severe than usual and make it more difficult to get to the doctor. Nevertheless, this visit may prevent the illness from getting worse. Here are some suggestions for getting to the doctor:

- Leave plenty of time to get to the appointment. You cannot hurry a person with Alzheimer's. Any pressure to hurry up usually results only in upset. Just try to keep the focus on getting ready to leave.
- Make sure that you are dressed and ready to leave before you start attending to your relative. It may be hard for him or her to wait for you.
- If your family member generally resists going to the doctor, do not mention the appointment before you get there. Instead, talk about something pleasant that you are going to do together, such as having lunch at a restaurant or visiting a friend.
- Try to bring another family member, a friend, or home health aide along to help you reassure or distract your relative.

- If your family member is in the moderate or moderately severe stage of AD, pack a bag with a change of clothes, incontinence products, and some activity to occupy him or her while you wait in the office. Just before you leave, include a snack and a drink.

WHAT SHOULD YOU DO WHEN YOU GET TO THE DOCTOR'S OFFICE?

Once you have gotten to the office, you will probably have to wait to see the doctor. Your relative may not be able to sit quietly until his or her turn, but may wander around, touch things that belong to other people, or talk with other patients who are not interested in a conversation. Don't become anxious or over-control your relative when these behaviors occur. In most cases, other people will not be as disturbed by your relative's behavior as you are. Instead, keep your relative occupied by looking at magazines together or eating the snack that you have brought along.

Do not be surprised if, when it is finally your turn to see the doctor, your relative refuses to go into the examining room. Although you may feel frustrated and embarrassed, it will probably not help to insist. People with AD may change their minds from moment to moment, so wait a few minutes and try again. A little later your relative may be willing to cooperate. If not, suggest a visit to the restroom, and afterwards move on to the examining room rather than return to the waiting room. If he or she still resists going into the examining room, the doctor may be willing to do the examination in a consultation room, which may be less frightening.

WHAT SHOULD YOU TELL THE DOCTOR?

Whether you are visiting for the first time or it is a return appointment, tell the doctor about any changes in your family member's behavior, since they may be a sign of physical illness. People with AD often are not able to say when or where they feel pain. If you think there have been changes in vision or hearing, discuss your concerns during routine visits to the doctor, who may recommend seeing a specialist.

If you have completed the *Profile of the Person with Memory Impairment,* use it as a reference. If not, make an accurate list or bring along all the bottles of medicine your relative takes to show the doctor.

WHAT IS YOUR ROLE WHEN YOUR RELATIVE IS BEING EXAMINED?

How much you participate depends on how able to cooperate and communicate your family member is. You will need to weigh sensitivity to your relative's self-esteem and wish for privacy against the doctor's need for accurate information and cooperation with the examination. Here are some questions to consider. Should your relative be asked what is bothering him or her or should you describe the problem? Should you go into the examination room with your family member? Should you help your relative with potentially difficult procedures such as providing a urine sample? Of course the answers to these questions depend on the severity of the dementia, your relationship with your family member, gender issues, and how comfortable you feel about helping with personal care.

If you are not able to be in the examining room, or feel uncomfortable with certain procedures, the nurse or your family member's home health aide, if there is one, may be able to help.

WHAT SHOULD YOU DO IF YOUR RELATIVE WILL NOT COOPERATE?

Once your relative is in the examination room, he or she may be calm and cooperative, and the rest of the appointment may go very well. If, on the other hand, he or she is upset and uncooperative, it can be very upsetting and embarrassing.

Remain calm. If you have taken time off from work or put a lot of effort into getting your family member to the doctor, you may feel particularly frustrated, defeated, and angry when he or she does not cooperate. Upon finding yourself getting tense and irritated, take a few deep breaths and make an effort to regain your composure. Remember that people with AD lose the ability to be flexible. Don't lose yours. A sense of humor may also help.

If your family member becomes agitated or extremely uncooperative, ask the doctor to perform only those procedures that will provide essential information. It may be hard for your relative to give a urine sample, get an injection, have blood drawn, or comply with numerous other procedures. Find out if there are alternate means of accomplishing these tasks; otherwise, you may have to try again at another time.

◆   ◆   ◆

Tony K realized that he had made a big mistake by telling his wife Brenda, who was in the moderately severe stage of AD, that they were going to the doctor the next day. He had promised himself that he wouldn't tell her about upcoming events. Although he had meant to reassure her with the information, he wound up upsetting her instead. Of course she was up all night going through her closet looking for something to wear and waking him up to ask if it was time to go. When it finally was time to get ready for the appointment, she was so agitated that she could not eat her breakfast and refused to take her regular medicine.

Tony was afraid that in her current state Brenda would not be able to cooperate with the doctor. He was not wrong. Getting urine and blood samples had even been a problem on Brenda's good days. Fortunately, Tony was prepared with a few strategies to help the doctor complete his examination and do the necessary tests. He brought soda and candy in a briefcase. As soon as they got to the office, he gave Brenda the soda. Sure enough, her diaper was soaking wet by the time the doctor needed a urine sample. The nurse was then able to get a specimen by wringing it out of the diaper. When it was time to take her blood, Tony gave Brenda the candies. She was so distracted by sorting and eating them that she didn't even realize the nurse had put a needle in her arm. By the time they left the doctor's office she was in a good mood, and Tony was very pleased with how he had handled the situation.

◆   ◆   ◆

Usually the doctor will be able to complete enough of the examination to identify the problem that has brought your relative to the office.

If you have chosen well, you can expect a reasonable amount of under-standing and patience from both the doctor and staff.

If, however, your relative is not able to cooperate at all and the visit is truly routine, try again on another day. One of the blessings of this terri-ble disease is that your relative probably will forget the examination soon after you leave. Life with a person with AD is often unpredictable. The next appointment may go very smoothly.

· 4 ·

Medication and Alzheimer's Disease

Most elderly people take at least one medication on a regular basis. Many are being treated for conditions such as diabetes and heart disease that require a specific diet or scheduled medication. When people have Alzheimer's disease, however, it can be difficult for them to understand and follow their doctor's orders. You are probably more aware than your relative of the importance of taking medication as it is prescribed.

Sometimes the consequences of missing a dose or eating the wrong food are not immediately obvious. But some medications must be taken on schedule, with or without food, and cannot be stopped abruptly. If you are responsible for making sure a family member with AD takes prescribed medicines, it is essential to do so without creating a crisis. This chapter will provide some helpful tips.

IN THIS CHAPTER

Do You Understand the Prescription?

What Is the Role of the Pharmacist in Medical Care?

How Can You Help Your Family Member Take Medicine and Follow a Teatment Plan?

Are There Special Medicines for Alzheimer's Disease?

DO YOU UNDERSTAND THE PRESCRIPTION?

After a visit to the doctor's office, you may receive a prescription for new medication or the refill of an old one. Be sure you understand what is being prescribed and how it is to be taken. A good idea is to write down this information or ask the doctor to do so. The directions should also be clearly stated on the label. If you are curious about the abbreviations on the prescription, see the Appendix at the back of this book. Do not be afraid to ask questions. If this is a new medication, double check with the doctor to be sure that it will not cause problems for an elderly person with dementia. Ask about possible side effects and what you should do if they develop. It is generally a bad idea to stop a medication abruptly, so find out in advance what you should do if your relative has a bad reaction to it, or accidentally misses or doubles up on a dose.

WHAT IS THE ROLE OF THE PHARMACIST IN MEDICAL CARE?

It is a good idea to fill all prescriptions at the same pharmacy, especially if your relative is being treated by more than one physician. A doctor may write a prescription without knowing all the other medicines your family member is taking, but if all prescriptions are filled at the same place, the pharmacist will have a complete record. This can be vital since medicines sometimes interfere with each other or even cause bad side effects when taken together. The pharmacist can be helpful in other ways as well. For example, many medicines come in more than one form. They may be available as liquids, pills, or powders. A pharmacist can tell you whether the medicine the doctor has prescribed comes in a form that is easier for a person with dementia to take. If so, have the pharmacist call the doctor to ask if it is possible to change the prescription.

Finally, pharmacists are knowledgeable about side effects and other medicine-related matters. They can answer many questions you might have forgotten or did not want to ask the doctor. It may also be easier to talk with someone in the neighborhood with whom you do not need to make an appointment.

◆ ◆ ◆

Mr. A had always been very careful about his medications. He knew exactly what he was taking and what it was for. When he and his daughter spoke on the phone recently, he told her that he had not been feeling well and was taking aspirins. "I don't think I handled this too well," his daughter admitted, "because I heard myself shrieking, 'Dad you know you can't take aspirin!'" In the most sheepish voice, Mr A asked what the problem was. "Everybody takes aspirin," he said. What he did not remember was that he had developed a serious bleeding problem in his stomach a few months earlier and was on doctor's orders not to take them.

"Even though my father seemed to be doing so well, I realized right then that I had to get more involved with his care. I didn't want to offend him— he takes such pride in caring for himself—but I knew I was going to have to clear out all but his essential medications and let his doctor know what had happened."

Even though Mr. A was in the mild stage of Alzheimer's, it had become clear to his daughter that he did not always understand or remember what was being said to him. She also realized how hard it was to find a delicate balance between caring and butting in.

◆　　◆　　◆

HOW CAN YOU HELP YOUR FAMILY MEMBER TAKE MEDICINE AND FOLLOW A TREATMENT PLAN?

People with AD may have trouble understanding or following instructions for taking medicine. They may forget to take it, or forget that they have taken it and take it again. People in the mild stage may deny or not be aware that they are having problems taking their medication, refilling prescriptions on time, and following their medical treatment plan. If they live alone, their family caregiver will have to find ways to make sure they are taking their medication safely. Here are some ideas that might help:

- Check empty medicine bottles or full ones, and look for dropped pills on the floor when you visit.
- Be alert to changes in mood or orientation when you speak to your relative on the phone.

- Be prepared to step in and provide more supervision before danger arises.

In the moderate and moderately severe stages of dementia, people sometimes get into a stubborn mood and simply refuse to take their medication, do their exercises, or follow a prescribed diet. Since missing a dose of medication or eating the wrong food can be very serious and sometimes lead to hospitalization or worse, it may be difficult for you not to react in an extreme way—either by trying to force your family member to cooperate or by withdrawing altogether, even though that may be dangerous. But a more complicated situation may occur late in the disease, when swallowing becomes difficult, and you will need to consult with the doctor on a safe way to give medicines to your relative.

If other people take care of your relative part of the time, be sure that they know the medication schedule, the diet to follow, and treatments to give. Make a list of all the medicines your relative must take and the times when they are to be taken and post it in an obvious place. Be sure all medicines are where they can be found by a responsible adult, but out of reach of the person with AD.

STRATEGIES FOR HELPING
YOUR FAMILY MEMBER TAKE MEDICINE

- Lay out the pills in a box that has sections marked for each time of day and each day of the week.
- Put the medicine next to your relative's plate at mealtime (especially if the medicine is to be taken with food and not on an empty stomach).
- Tell your family member that he or she can have something special, like a cookie, after taking the medicine.
- Ask the pharmacist if it is okay to disguise the pill by grinding it into a powder and putting it into a food with a strong flavor.
- If your relative has trouble swallowing pills, ask the doctor to prescribe medicine in liquid form.

- If your family member refuses to take the medicine, wait a few minutes and try again.
- If he or she won't take the medicine from you, ask someone else to try. Your relative may react differently to another person.
- Say the doctor called to ask if the medication has been taken, and you need to call back with an answer.
- While your family member is engaged in another activity, calmly hand over the medication in a matter-of-fact way.

When a person with dementia no longer understands why it is important to follow a special diet or do his or her exercises, you may become angry because you are aware of the consequences. It is hard to have to say, "No, you can't have cake," or "You have to do your range-of-motion exercises." The general idea is to focus in a positive way on the behavior or activity you want to encourage. This approach can reduce the stress on you and your relative at the same time it creates opportunities for pleasant experiences for both of you. Consider the following suggestions:

- Try to keep foods your relative is not supposed to have out of sight. Do not eat them or serve them to others when your relative is present, unless you have a substitute for him or her. In short, try to say, "Yes, you can have this," instead of, "No, you can't have that."
- Invite your family member to participate, rather than demand that he or she do so.
- When it is time to do exercises, put on some music and start doing them yourself. Your relative may catch your positive mood and join in the fun.

◆   ◆   ◆

Until recently, Mrs. J was very easygoing about taking her medicine. It had become a regular part of her routine, and she would look for her dish of pills when dessert was served. Suddenly she began to put up a fuss. She wanted to know what each pill was for, and insisted that she had never taken pills before and was not going to start now. When this first started happening, her husband got very upset and went into a long explanation, trying to convince her that it was important for her health to take her medicine regularly. All that accomplished was to make her walk out of the room.

"Now I wait a little while after dinner, bring the dish of pills to her, and ask in a casual way if she is ready to take them. She usually agrees. And when she doesn't take them right away, I just wait a while and ask again."

Mrs. J's moods change pretty quickly, so Mr. J does not worry or try to lecture her anymore. He also has a few other tricks up his sleeve that he learned from the people in his support group. "Some of them grind up the pills and put them in something like applesauce, but we are not there yet."

♦   ♦   ♦

ARE THERE SPECIAL MEDICATIONS FOR ALZHEIMER'S DISEASE?

Currently there are no medications that will cure AD or reverse damage already done, but some can now reduce symptoms and possibly slow the progression of the illness. They seem to be effective at the mild and moderate stages. If you have questions about whether these medications would be suitable for your family member, ask his or her primary care physician, neurologist, or geriatric psychiatrist.

Other medications are sometimes prescribed to relieve symptoms of Alzheimer's disease such as anxiety, depression, agitation, hallucinations, and delusions. They can be effective, but must be used with caution and monitored by a knowledgeable physician since they may have unwanted side effects. Use of these medications should be reviewed regularly, since some symptoms such as paranoia or agitation may decrease or go away entirely as the disease progresses.

Some symptoms of dementia—such as incontinence, physical rigidity, or poor balance—cannot currently be treated with medications. In many cases, however, it is possible to relieve these and other symptoms by making changes in the environment or in the way the person is cared for rather than by using medications.

CLINICAL TRIALS

What Is a Clinical Drug Trial?

New drugs are being developed all the time for AD as well as other diseases. Before they can be put on the market, though, they must be tested on many people under strict scientific conditions and approved by the Federal Food and Drug Administration (FDA).

Drug companies usually first turn to medical centers and later to doctors in the community to conduct clinical trials of new medications. They need to know if the drug is safe and if it works, as well as if there are any side effects and how serious they may be. In most cases, research subjects are given drugs that have already been extensively tested to be sure they will not cause patients any serious harm.

Most clinical trials are set up so that some participants (the treatment or experimental group) receive the drug, while some (the control group) are given an inactive substance or a placebo. This helps the researchers know if changes in the patient are due to the drug rather than to other factors, such as the belief that the medication will help (known as the *placebo effect*). In a double-blind, placebo-controlled study, no one—not the patient, family, doctor, or researchers—knows which group the patient is in. Sometimes subjects who have been receiving the placebo will, after a period of time, be offered the chance to receive the active medication.

There are also other important kinds of studies that do not involve drugs or may include testing a medication in combination with an activity program such as exercise, group support, or counseling. In all these studies, participants contribute to the advancement of knowledge about the disease and the development of improved methods of treatment. They also have the chance to benefit from the latest medical and psychological advances and to receive the best medical care available.

Should Your Family Member Take Part in a Clinical Trial?

If your relative is no longer able to make medical decisions, it will be up to you to decide whether or not to enroll him or her in a study.

This decision, like many others you make for your relative, should be based on what you believe he or she would have wanted and what you think is best. You should also consider the extra responsibilities you will have to take on if your family member joins a study, and what benefits you can expect. You or your relative, if he or she is able, will be asked to sign a document called an *informed consent,* which states that the person signing understands the purpose and risks of the trial and accepts the obligations of participating.

Do not hesitate to ask questions so you can make an informed decision. Those that follow will help you decide whether or not you want to enroll your family member in a particular study.

- What is the purpose of the study?
- Is this the kind of study in which some people don't get the drug being tested?
- How long will it last?
- What will your relative be expected to do? Will he or she have to take medication, take part in an activity, etc.?
- What does your relative need to do to qualify? Take medical and/or cognitive tests, discontinue certain medications, make repeated visits to the clinic, etc.?
- How many visits are involved? How long will they last? Can somebody other than you bring your family member?
- What are the potential risks involved in joining the study? What are the potential benefits?
- Will there be someone to call if you have a question or a problem?

Clinical trials have very strict rules (called *criteria*) about who can participate, such as the stage of the patient's disease and other medical conditions. If your relative applies for a clinical trial and he or she is not accepted, you may be very disappointed, but you should not be insulted or feel that your relative has "failed a test" or done something "wrong."

Subjects in clinical trials may get the opportunity to benefit from the newest treatments and be examined frequently to chart their progress and pick up any problems. There is never a financial cost for participating in research, and sometimes an allowance is provided for transportation, parking, and food.

How can you find out about clinical trials in your area? Ask your doctor or support group leader, call the Alzheimer's Association or nearest Alzheimer's Disease Center, or look on the Internet. The National Institutes of Health has a web site (www.clinicaltrials.gov) that gives general information about clinical trials, and lists all trials according to disease. This is a good place to start.

◆ 5 ◆

Mental Health Care for a Person with Alzheimer's Disease

Since Alzheimer's disease is not a mental but a physical illness that destroys parts of the brain, it has an impact on all aspects of an individual's life and health, including emotional well-being. It is understandable for those diagnosed to be worried about the immediate effects this illness will have on them and their families, and what it will mean in the future. As the disease progresses, they will need a great deal of emotional support to hold on to a sense of personal worth in the face of increasing disability. They will also need their environments to be modified and simplified to enable them to function at their best.

IN THIS CHAPTER

How Can You Help Your Family Member Maintain Emotional Well-Being?

Should You Tell Your Family Member That He or She Has Alzheimer's Disease?

Should Others Be Told That Your Relative Has Alzheimer's Disease?

Are There Things You Should Not Tell Your Relative?

What Kinds of Activities Can Improve the Emotional Well-Being of People with Alzheimer's Disease?

Is There Treatment for People with Alzheimer's Disease Who Are Depressed?
What Can You Do about Your Relative's Disturbing Behavior?
Where Can You Go for Help?

HOW CAN YOU HELP YOUR FAMILY MEMBER MAINTAIN EMOTIONAL WELL-BEING?

Although it is not currently possible to stop the progression of the illness itself, many of the painful emotional reactions and behavioral disturbances that often accompany Alzheimer's disease can be relieved. These are symptoms that should not be ignored. They frequently make life more unpleasant, add to the disability of AD sufferers, and cause them to appear more demented.

Since such people are easily confused and upset when there is too much going on, caregivers should be aware of particularly stressful situations and know how to create an environment that will enable their family member to function at the highest possible level. Perhaps the most effective thing you can do to help your family member feel confident and safe is to modify the home so that it remains appropriate for his or her changing needs and abilities.

- Simplify the surroundings while keeping them as familiar as possible.
- Remove unnecessary objects so that your relative will have less trouble finding what he or she needs. (Since people with Alzheimer's often put other people's possessions away in strange places, it may save you time and aggravation if you put them out of the way yourself.)
- Make sure there is adequate lighting because shadows and dark places may be frightening to someone with AD.
- Only rearrange furniture when necessary—to create clear pathways around the room and from one room to another.
- Replace complicated appliances with simpler ones to prevent feelings of frustration. (A radio with one or two knobs can be used more easily than one with many controls.)

In addition to dealing with the physical surroundings, there are other ways to contribute to your relative's well-being, such as maintaining a regular daily routine, since it is hard for people with AD to adjust to new situations and places. Knowing what to expect will help him or her feel more in control and less dependent on you and others for information about what is going to happen next.

Also, try to avoid saying things that may make your family member feel bad about him or herself. For example, when you get frustrated because he or she does not remember what you have repeated many times, you may feel like saying, "I told you that before," or "How many times do I have to tell you that?" This can be very hurtful to a person who cannot remember. Rather than lose your patience, make a joke out of it, pretend you yourself forgot and repeat it one more time, or change the subject.

People with AD are particularly sensitive to being rushed or ordered around. If you are calm and supportive, and understand what your relative can and cannot do, he or she may have greater self-esteem and feel less depressed or anxious. For instance, do not rely on him or her to give people messages or take them when answering the phone. If the last time you asked your relative to hold something for you, it was lost, don't make him or her responsible for valuable items.

Many people with AD are afraid to be alone and will follow a familiar person around the house. It may help to give your relative something to do that will keep him or her occupied while having you in sight. Try to make sure your relative is alone as little as possible.

DEFINITIONS

Anxiety: A feeling of worry or fear, which frequently causes restlessness.

Depression: A mood disturbance marked by sadness and feelings of worthlessness or hopelessness.

Neither of these conditions is unique to Alzheimer's disease, but both can be caused or made worse by it.

SHOULD YOU TELL YOUR FAMILY MEMBER THAT HE OR SHE HAS ALZHEIMER'S DISEASE?

One of the first decisions you may face is whether or not to tell your family member that he or she has been diagnosed with Alzheimer's disease. There is no single right answer to this question. Some professionals believe it is their ethical obligation to inform their patient, others prefer to decide on an individual basis after consultation with the family, and still others feel it is never appropriate to tell an AD patient about the diagnosis.

A reasonable approach may be to give your relative a little bit of information, see what the reaction is, and then provide some more information if you think he or she will be able to tolerate it. This way of dealing with potentially upsetting information may be useful in other situations as well.

◆　　◆　　◆

Denise G was really concerned about her mother finding out that she had Alzheimer's. She asked every doctor who took care of her mother to use the term memory problem. *But then the neurologist who was part of the team that did the formal cognitive evaluation on Mrs. G, said in her mother's presence that the tests had ruled out everything except Alzheimer's disease.*

"I thought that was a pretty cagey way of telling her without actually saying that she had Alzheimer's," Denise said. "I was surprised and relieved that my mother did not appear to understand the implication of his explanation, and she has never used this term in relation to herself.

"I think it is very curious that my mother keeps picking up articles about Alzheimer's disease and saying that she thinks this is what's wrong with my father." Still, Mrs. G has never mentioned her own meeting with the neurologist, and when Denise has tried to talk to her about it, she just changes the subject.

"I guess I'm not in denial anymore, but my mother still is. Maybe her comments about my father are her way of talking about herself. Still, her attitude makes things hard for me since this is something important that we can't discuss."

◆　　◆　　◆

People in the mild stage of Alzheimer's may be able to understand the meaning of the diagnosis and want to make plans for their future. They may choose to participate in activities designed especially for people with AD, such as early patient support groups. In this situation, the person can benefit from being informed. Sometimes people who are told the diagnosis when they are at an early stage "choose" not to hear it, which may be their way of protecting themselves from uncomfortable information they would rather not have. If this is the case with your relative, it is best not to press further.

Because of the nature of the disease, even people who appear to know they have AD may sometimes forget that they do. They may not realize that they are having problems or that the problems they are having can be explained by the disease. Eventually the progression of the disease makes the issue of whether or not to tell irrelevant because people in later stages can no longer remember the diagnosis or recognize its impact on them.

♦   ♦   ♦

"I really wish my family had not been so ashamed when my dad got sick. We tried to hide things as long as we could, but I think people knew and just didn't say anything," said George H. His family had been reluctant to talk about the changes they all noticed in his father, and no one was facing the need to make plans for the future. George saw that there was another way of handling it when he got together with his cousins.

"We were sitting together at a wedding, and they talked openly about their mother, my Aunt Jean, being diagnosed with Alzheimer's disease. She was right there with them and joined in the discussion." His cousins spoke of their plans to fix up Jean's apartment, enroll in support groups, and meet with an elder care lawyer to make financial arrangements. "It was such a relief to be able to talk freely. I hoped I could convince my family to do the same."

♦   ♦   ♦

SHOULD OTHERS BE TOLD YOUR RELATIVE HAS ALZHEIMER'S DISEASE?

Families approach this decision from many different points of view. Some feel that the longer they are able to conceal the diagnosis, the longer their relative will be treated or behave "normally." Some prefer to let others know promptly in the hope that their relative will receive more understanding and support.

Whatever decision you make in regard to family and friends, it is always important to let doctors and other medical personnel know about the diagnosis. It will help them, with your input, to provide the best care for your family member with AD.

ARE THERE THINGS YOU SHOULD NOT TELL YOUR RELATIVE?

You may find yourself working overtime to avoid subjects that will upset your relative. This adds to your burden by putting unreasonable demands on you. Since Alzheimer's disease can last for many years, it is likely that many important events will have occurred in the world at large as well as within the family during that time. Especially in the early stages of the illness, you will not be able to control what your family member hears, reads, or is told by other people. Even if you could do this, it would not always be possible to know in advance what information will prove to be upsetting.

Sometimes even good or happy news can be stressful for a person with AD. He or she may share the excitement about an upcoming family wedding, for example, but become very concerned about what to wear, how to get there, and then be confused about who is on which side of the family. In situations like this, it is a good idea to always have someone by your relative's side to provide cues and reassurance.

When told about the death of a family member or close friend, your relative with AD may become agitated or anxious and behave in ways that seem inappropriate, like seeming not to care, forgetting the person has died, or getting confused about who has died. Although this may disturb you, try to remember that these reactions are caused by your relative's dementia.

How can you decide what to tell a person with Alzheimer's? Does he or she have a right to know about something even if it might be very upsetting? If his or her sister dies, for example, should your relative be told? This is an ethical dilemma constantly faced by caregivers of people with dementia. While you want to avoid unnecessarily placing your family member in difficult situations, you don't want to leave him or her out of the life of the family. Here are some questions to help you decide what to do.

- Is your relative able to understand the situation?
- Will he or she remember the information?
- How has he or she responded to similar situations in the recent past?
- Will you be able to handle a negative reaction?

If you think you may be upset or frightened by your relative's response to bad news, and you feel the need to tell him or her nevertheless, plan how to deal with the reaction in advance. Enlist the support of family, friends, or other people you rely on (such as a minister, social worker, or physician).

WHAT KINDS OF ACTIVITIES CAN IMPROVE THE EMOTIONAL WELL-BEING OF PEOPLE WITH ALZHEIMER'S DISEASE?

As Alzheimer's progresses, your relative will be less able to participate in the activities that used to fill the day and provide interest and satisfaction, such as working, visiting with friends, and engaging in a hobby. He or she will require more help to structure time and find things to do to relieve what has been called the *empty day syndrome*. This constant need for company and direction leaves many caregivers feeling trapped.

You can find simple chores for your family member to do at home. Depending on the stage of the disease, having him or her help with food preparation, simple cleaning, folding laundry, and gardening may be possible. Even if this is not actually very helpful to you, it is important that your relative still feel like a contributor to family life.

He or she may still enjoy watching television and listening to music. Sometimes, however, when people have reached the moderate stage of AD, they have trouble telling the difference between the images on television and real life. They may believe that the people on the screen are actually in the house and look for them, become frightened, or think they have to play host to "visitors." When your relative reaches this stage, you should carefully choose the TV programs or rent appropriate videos.

There are videos made especially for people with Alzheimer's (see Appendix), where the person on the screen invites the viewer to join with him or her in singing popular songs or asks simple questions to which the person can respond. As always, your knowledge of your relative will help you choose the programs that are most likely to be of interest.

Adult day care programs provide structured activities such as music, exercise, crafts, trips, and discussions, as well as opportunities for socializing in a safe environment (some day care centers also offer medical care) geared to the physical and mental abilities of a person with dementia. These programs are best suited for people with moderate AD. Although it may be hard for you to accept that your family member has reached this stage of dementia, participating in activities at a day care center is likely to enhance his or her mood and sense of belonging. Some of these services are covered by Medicaid. Others require payment, often on a sliding scale.

Senior centers, churches, Y's, and other social service organizations may also offer programs that are suitable for someone with AD. You may even find an activity you can go to together. Several organizations have volunteers who will visit a person with AD, while students training to work with the elderly may also want the experience of learning about the disease. Your relative may become their "teacher," making the exchange valuable to everyone concerned.

IS THERE TREATMENT FOR PEOPLE WITH ALZHEIMER'S DISEASE WHO ARE DEPRESSED?

Symptoms of depression frequently occur in the mild and moderate stages of Alzheimer's disease. There are several possible reasons for this. Many people become very sad when they recognize that they have a serious, chronic illness that has damaged their memory. Others are reluctant to be in social situations because they are embarrassed by their forgetfulness, and become depressed from being alone too much.

People with dementia may be apathetic (uninterested in things) and passive or withdrawn. They may move slowly and speak less often. They may also become tearful and even say they want to die. Experts disagree about whether these symptoms are due to Alzheimer's disease itself or a psychological depression. If they last for more than a few weeks, you should seek advice from a physician. Whatever the cause, depression in AD can be effectively treated with medications that are particularly suitable for an elderly person with dementia.

Emotional support may also be very helpful at this time. Support groups for people in the mild stage of AD are now widely available. They provide companionship and the opportunity to hear how other people are coping with their illness. By reducing isolation and increasing self-esteem, these groups can help relieve depression. If you believe your family member is embarrassed by his or her disabilities and is withdrawing from regular social activities, try to find less challenging social situations or activities geared toward people with memory impairment or dementia. Although it is not yet common practice, individual psychotherapy with a therapist who has experience treating people with AD, either in combination with medicine or by itself, can be very beneficial.

WHAT CAN YOU DO ABOUT YOUR RELATIVE'S DISTURBING BEHAVIOR?

Beginning in the moderate stage, your family member may behave in peculiar ways and experience a variety of psychiatric symptoms such as insomnia, agitation, hallucinations, delusions, and paranoia. It may be useful to think about these symptoms, which are probably due both to the brain changes of AD and the confusion it causes, as your relative's way of communicating, even if the message is not clear. Try to understand what he or she needs and respond as best you can. Your efforts may even reduce or eliminate the peculiar behavior while also showing respect for your family member's dignity.

Some of these symptoms, such as delusions (where a person believes things that are not true) and hallucinations (where he or she sees or hears things that are not there), can be very upsetting to both of you. If your relative becomes frightened by something that is not there, make it clear that you are not afraid and will keep him or her safe. Distracting or taking him or her to another room may also work. But do not contradict, argue, or insist that he or she is wrong, because that will only make matters worse.

Sometimes, however, the delusion or hallucination is of a pleasant experience. When this happens, you do not need to do anything about it. Nor do you have to say that you can see or hear the same thing. Just be glad that something pleasant is occupying your family member's mind.

Try to identify what brings on disturbing behavior. If there is something in the environment, the activity, or the way you talk to your family member that seems to provoke this behavior, you may be able to change or avoid it.

If symptoms become too frightening or threatening for you to handle, do not be ashamed to ask for help. It may be worthwhile to consult with a geriatric psychiatrist, who can select a suitable treatment combining behavior management strategies and medications. A short hospitalization may sometimes be necessary to provide a safe environment until the proper dose of medication is selected and has time to take effect.

WHERE CAN YOU GO FOR HELP?

In addition to physicians, there are also many other resources for people with AD and their families. Your local chapter of the Alzheimer's Association can direct you to support groups for both patients and caregivers, and also refer you to adult day care programs suitable for people in the moderate stage. Social service organizations and religious and community centers often have programs for people with dementia, while some assisted living facilities and nursing homes provide respite services. Your relative will be able to stay there anywhere from a few days to a few weeks and receive appropriate care if you want to go away, are ill, or need a rest. There are also books, videotapes, web sites, support groups, and organizations that can help. See the section on Resources in the Appendix.

· 6 ·

Who Will Make Medical Decisions for a Person with Alzheimer's Disease?

If you have been caring for a person with Alzheimer's disease for a long time, you have probably found yourself making more and more decisions. Some seem to come naturally, without any special thought. You guide your relative through everyday activities, make appointments, may even decide what he or she wears and eats. When it comes to health care, though, the issues usually are much more complex, and the outcome of the decisions you make can be more serious and far reaching. This chapter looks at your role in medical decision making for a person with AD and offers some strategies to help you feel that you are doing what is best.

IN THIS CHAPTER

Can People with Alzheimer's Disease Make Medical Decisions for Themselves?

Should You Include Your Family Member in Making Medical Decisions?

What Are Advance Directives?

Who Can Help You Make Medical Decisions for Your Relative?

CAN PEOPLE WITH ALZHEIMER'S DISEASE MAKE MEDICAL DECISIONS FOR THEMSELVES?

Some people believe that older adults cannot make medical decisions on their own. This is not true. Many people remain mentally sound for their entire lives or at least well into old age. Older adults have both the life experience and the right to make decisions about what affects them. For people with Alzheimer's disease, however, medical decision making is much more complicated, since they gradually lose the ability to understand new information and think rationally. Still, they have rights as individuals and will continue to have those rights as long as they live.

In the mild stage of the illness, a person may have fairly serious memory problems but still be able to express a preference for a certain kind of treatment. This preference should be followed if at all possible. Even in the later stages, a person who has not voluntarily given someone else permission to make decisions on his or her behalf still has the legal right to continue to make them. Only a formal court procedure, which rarely occurs, can limit a person's autonomy. What generally happens is that as the disease progresses and the person with AD is no longer able to function independently, the family caregiver will have to make more of the decisions.

SHOULD YOU INCLUDE YOUR FAMILY MEMBER IN MAKING MEDICAL DECISIONS?

There are no hard and fast rules to tell you exactly how much you can rely on your family member to make an intelligent or responsible choice when it comes to medical decisions. Nonetheless, it is important to try to include a person with AD in the decision-making process as much as possible. Even when the dementia is quite advanced, there are still some choices the affected person can make if they are explained in simple terms.

Sometimes a person with AD understands the options, makes a choice, and then forgets that the discussion ever took place. Still, having had the discussion may be enough to make you feel comfortable that you are following your relative's wishes.

◆   ◆   ◆

Gloria's mother, Mrs. E, repeatedly complained that her eye was bothering her. Gloria took her mother to the eye doctor, who told Mrs. E that her eyelid was drooping and this might be causing her discomfort. He also explained that the droop could be surgically repaired, and gave her the name of an eye surgeon. Gloria listened with distress as her mother eagerly took the surgeon's card and seemed intent on having the operation, contrary to her usual behavior. Although Mrs. E understood that something could be done, she was not able to consider the risks of anesthesia to someone like herself. Gloria was also afraid that her mother, in the moderate stage of AD, would not be able to comply with the aftercare instructions.

When they got home, Gloria told her mother that although the decision was up to her, any surgery was dangerous, and if she could tolerate things as they were, it would be best to leave well enough alone. Her mother quickly agreed, although Gloria was positive the subject would come up again. She planned to use the same argument the next time, since she was sure that her mother, despite not remembering having had the discussion, would come to the same conclusion. It comforted Gloria to know that it was actually her mother's own wishes that were being fulfilled.

◆   ◆   ◆

If you know the person well and have discussed what he or she would want in advance, it will be easier to make decisions when the time comes. That is why you should talk about the medical care he or she will want later on while your relative is still in the mild stage of the illness.

People with dementia may live for many years after they are no longer able to make decisions for themselves. It is important for their family caregivers to know if they want to be kept alive at all costs or whether they would prefer only comfort or palliative care. Although it may be painful to discuss these issues, doing so means you will be able to follow your relative's wishes when he or she is no longer able to express them. These decisions should be formalized in documents called *advance directives*.

If your relative has prepared them, naming you health care proxy, your authority to make medical decisions for him or her will always be recognized. If there are no written instructions, most doctors will consult family members about medical decisions for cognitively impaired patients with dementia. Problems can occur, however, when family members do not agree and the patient has not expressed his or her wishes in writing.

WHAT ARE ADVANCE DIRECTIVES?

The right to voluntarily delegate another person to make certain decisions for you is recognized throughout the United States. In the past these arrangements only took care of financial and legal matters. Now they are made for personal and health care decision making as well.

Advance directives are written legal documents intended to tell family, friends, doctors, and other concerned professionals what an individual's wishes are for care when he or she can no longer express them. Advance directives may be needed in situations ranging from a sudden injury or illness to end-of-life care. Anyone can express these wishes, and all of us should do so, in writing, before an emergency arises.

There are two basic kinds of advance directives: power of attorney and living will. Powers of attorney appoint someone to make decisions (financial, legal) for people who cannot or do not want to make them for themselves, living wills state the kind of medical treatment people want or do not want when they can no longer declare their wishes, and some documents combine these two instruments.

Each of these directives has a different purpose. They differ in the circumstances they cover, when they go into effect, how they can be cancelled or changed, whether they require a lawyer to draft them, and whether they need to be witnessed or notarized. The needs of the individual and the laws of the state in which your relative lives will determine the most appropriate one. Resources for additional information about advance directives are listed in the Appendix.

Some of the life-sustaining treatments about which people need to state their care preference include artificial nutrition and hydration, and cardiopulmonary resuscitation.

Since, in the case of dementia, the inability to make decisions is predictable, these documents should be discussed and completed when people with AD are still able to express their thoughts and feelings about the medical care they want, so that if you are named proxy, you can

DEFINITIONS

Advance directive: A written document that tells what health care treatments a person wants or does not want when he or she cannot make these wishes known.

Artificial nutrition and hydration: When synthetic food (or nutrients) and water are fed to a person from a tube inserted through the nose into the stomach, directly into the intestine, or into a vein.

Comfort care: Care that helps to keep a person comfortable but does not cure the disease. Bathing, turning, keeping the lips and mouth moist, and pain medications are examples of comfort care.

Cardiopulmonary resuscitation (CPR): Treatment to try and restart a person's breathing or heartbeat. CPR may be done by breathing into the mouth, pushing on the chest, putting a tube through the mouth or nose into the throat, administering medication, giving electric shock to the chest, or by other means.

Durable power of attorney for health care: A document that appoints a specific individual to make health care decisions for a person who is unable to make them.

Life-sustaining treatment: Any medical treatment that is used to delay the moment of death. A breathing machine (ventilator), CPR, and artificial nutrition and hydration are examples of life-sustaining treatments.

Living will: Instructions made in advance that tell what medical treatment a person unable to make his or her wishes known does or does not want.

Permanent vegetative state: When a person is unconscious and has no hope of regaining consciousness even with medical treatment.

Surrogate decision maker (or health care proxy or agent): This is an individual, organization, or other body authorized to make health care decisions for a person unable to do so.

make the health care decisions the person whose proxy you are would have wanted.

All advance directives need to be written and signed while the individual whose wishes are being expressed is still able to understand them. If your family member is already in the hospital and has not made advance directives, the patient representative may be able to help you draw up these documents.

Since laws regarding advance directives are not the same in every state, you should find out what is required in the state where your relative lives. According to federal law, if someone has come from another state and the forms have been prepared according to the laws in that state, they must be honored wherever the person is currently residing.

Although you may feel more comfortable having a lawyer draw up these documents, it is not necessary to do so. You can buy standard forms in a stationery or office supply store, and get more information about advance directives from the American Geriatrics Society and the American Academy of Family Physicians (see Appendix).

Advance directives should be kept where they can easily be found, given to the person's doctor and the person named as the decision maker (called the *proxy*), and put in the patient's chart if he or she is hospitalized. If you have prepared a *crisis kit* (described in Chapter 8), a copy should be included in it.

WHO CAN HELP YOU MAKE MEDICAL DECISIONS FOR YOUR RELATIVE?

Of course, you can never make every decision in advance. Situations will arise that you cannot have expected. You may be torn between wanting more tests and treatment for your relative, and feeling that it is time to step back and let nature take its course.

If you are uncomfortable making these decisions despite being the designated proxy, involve other family members, or get help from clergy, your relative's doctor, or someone else whose opinion you trust. In the hospital, the social worker, patient representative, clergy, and ethics committee can help you make the appropriate decisions.

PART TWO

◆　　◆　　◆

Preparing for a
Hospitalization

◆ 7 ◆

The Profile of the Person with Memory Impairment

Every individual is unique. We each have likes and dislikes, interests and life experiences, abilities and disabilities, or other special needs. Most of us can express these details about ourselves. We certainly can tell people our address, phone number, and other important personal data; but people with Alzheimer's disease are generally less able to do so, and eventually cannot do so at all.

One of the most important steps a caregiver can take is to write down vital information about a family member with AD. Then there will be a permanent and accessible record of all the details that a person may no longer be able to provide, but which can make a big difference when he or she needs medical care.

IN THIS CHAPTER

What Is the *Profile of the Person with Memory Impairment?*

Who Should Use the *Profile of the Person with Memory Impairment?*

How Can the *Profile of the Person with Memory Impairment* Be Used?

WHAT IS THE *PROFILE OF*
THE *PERSON WITH MEMORY IMPAIRMENT?**

The *Profile of the Person with Memory Impairment* is a form designed to describe your family member quickly and clearly to anyone who will be taking care of him or her. It gives details about the way that person functions—if he or she can dress, bathe, and feed him or herself, walk without assistance, and understand instructions. Equally important, it will tell people who do not know your relative what kinds of situations are likely to be upsetting and the best strategies to calm him or her down. It contains questions you are best able to answer about day-to-day situations in the life of your family member, and also includes:

- Emergency contact information.
- A section describing interests, activities, and normal daily routine.
- Medical history.
- A list of medications normally taken (prescribed and over the counter).
- Allergies to food and medications.

Once you have filled out the *Profile*, the important details about your family member with AD will be written down, and you will not have to worry about forgetting to tell them to a doctor or other health care professional. Also, in case your family member has to be taken to the doctor by someone who does not know him or her as well as you do, the information will be available and can be passed along.

◆   ◆   ◆

While walking arm in arm with her paid companion to the senior center, Mrs. K tripped and fell. The aide called an ambulance. The good news is that a list of her medications—her doctor's name and phone number, the numbers of other family members, her date of birth, Social Security number, and insurance information—was posted on the wall at her home. Her

---

*Some caregivers prefer to use the term memory impairment rather than Alzheimer's disease on material that will be seen by their ill relative. That is why the form is entitled *Profile of a Person with Memory Impairment*. However, it is always best to give the actual diagnosis to those who treat or care for your relative *daughter Sally had also reviewed with the aide what to do in an emergency. The bad news is that the aide did not have a copy of the instructions with her when she left the house with Mrs. K.*

The aide asked the ambulance driver to stop at Mrs. K's house to get the list, so everything turned out okay. The lesson Sally learned was that it is important to have multiple copies of this information—in the aide's purse, in Mrs. K's pocket, and with every member of Mrs. K's family involved in her care.

◆ ◆ ◆

WHO SHOULD USE THE *PROFILE OF THE PERSON WITH MEMORY IMPAIRMENT*?

Even the most organized caregiver can forget important details in the midst of a medical emergency. It usually gets very chaotic when a person with AD requires medical care. The *Profile* will serve as a reminder of important information that you may forget under stress.

In addition, caregivers worry about what will happen if they are unavailable: if they become ill themselves and need to go to the hospital or are suddenly called away on urgent business. In such situations, it is a comfort to know that somebody else can use the information in the *Profile* to take good care of the person with AD. It should be kept in an obvious place in your relative's home, and everyone who spends time with him or her should have a copy. That way, other family members, a neighbor, or a home health aide will know what to do if you are not available to tell them yourself.

HOW CAN THE *PROFILE OF THE PERSON WITH MEMORY IMPAIRMENT* BE USED?

The *Profile* will be extremely useful to the medical staff in an emergency room or if a hospital admission is necessary. It will alert medical personnel that your relative has dementia and needs special care, and enable them to understand your relative's limitations so they can provide treatment in the most appropriate way.

The *Profile* has many other potential uses. For example, you should give a copy of it to your family member's primary care physician and other health care providers. It will be a ready reference about your relative's level of functioning, and a record of changes over time. If you are being interviewed by an intake worker at an adult day care program or at another service for your family member, much of the information in the *Profile* will be valuable. And if your relative spends time in such a setting, a copy should be available to all staff members there.

So be sure to take the time to complete the form. Photocopy the *Profile* in the Appendix of this book and fill in all the blanks as well as you can. Then make plenty of copies of the completed form, including a copy:

- For the crisis kit (see Chapter 8).
- To post near the phone in your relative's home.
- For each person who spends time with your family member.
- For yourself.

It is essential to update the *Profile* whenever there is a change in your family member's level of functioning, medical condition, or medications.

◆ 8 ◆

Planning Before the Crisis Comes

It is impossible to know when a medical crisis will occur, but when you are caring for a person with Alzheimer's disease, even an expected hospitalization can feel like a crisis. Planning in advance will reduce the stress on you in an emergency and make it easier for both you and your relative to get through the experience. This chapter will look at some strategies that will help if a hospitalization is necessary.

IN THIS CHAPTER

What Is a Crisis Kit?

Who Will Go to the Hospital with Your Relative If You Are Not Available?

Who Will Stay with Your Relative in the Hospital?

What Should You Ask Your Relative's Doctor in Advance?

What Should You Know about the Hospital?

What Will the Insurance Company Require?

What if You Are Caring for More Than One Disabled Person?

What Else Can You Plan in Advance?

WHAT IS A CRISIS KIT?

A crisis kit contains the necessary documents and personal belongings your relative will need if it becomes necessary to go to the hospital. You can avoid a mad scramble at the last minute if you have a bag already packed. It may make you feel uncomfortable to do this when your family member is not sick, but if there is a medical emergency, you will be glad you did it in advance. Not only that, but the crisis kit will make it easier for anyone else to take your family member to the hospital in an emergency.

WHAT INFORMATION
SHOULD BE IN THE CRISIS KIT?

- Your relative's Social Security and Medicare numbers. Details about additional medical insurance, including the name of the carrier and the policy number. A photocopy of insurance cards.
- Your relative's date of birth and address.
- The names of several people to contact in an emergency if you are not available.
- Copies of advance directives (see Chapter 6).
- The completed *Profile of the Person with Memory Impairment* (see Chapter 7).
- A copy of your family member's most recent EKG (electrocardiogram); ask the primary care physician to give you a copy for this purpose.
- A list of medications and dosages. This list should include everything your family member takes, prescription and over the counter. It is especially important to list vitamins and any herbal or nutritional supplements. Often medical personnel are not told about these substances, which can interact with other medicines, affect response to anesthesia, and cause symptoms such as headaches, dizziness, and weakness. All this information should be included in the *Profile,* but you may wish to have a separate list in the kit as well.

Put all this information in an envelope or folder marked with your family member's name and the words **Important Information** in bold letters.

WHAT PERSONAL ITEMS SHOULD BE IN THE CRISIS KIT?

- Bathrobe and slippers.
- Toiletries (toothbrush, toothpaste, cosmetics, soap, shampoo, etc.).
- Incontinence products.
- Containers for glasses, hearing aid, dentures, etc.
- Something to keep your relative occupied, such as a magazine or portable radio.
- A picture of a familiar person or place that has meaning to your relative.
- A few dollars to buy a newspaper, magazine, or refreshment, which will contribute to your relative's feeling of self-esteem.

Do not put anything valuable or expensive in the kit, such as jewelry, watches, or other items that might be distressing to lose. Put your relative's name on all personal items.

WHO WILL GO TO THE HOSPITAL WITH YOUR FAMILY MEMBER IF YOU ARE NOT AVAILABLE?

It is important to arrange in advance for someone to go to the hospital with your family member if you cannot. Ideally, this person will live nearby and know your relative well. Having a crisis kit ready will be especially useful in this situation. Make sure whoever is on standby knows where the crisis kit is, what it contains, and how to get in touch with you or another family member as soon as possible.

If the information about medical decisions that have been made for your relative (the kind included in advance directives) is contained in the crisis kit, whoever takes your relative to the hospital will have access to it and be able to convey it to the appropriate hospital personnel.

WHO WILL STAY WITH YOUR RELATIVE IN THE HOSPITAL?

People who suffer from dementia need a great deal of supervision and personal care in the hospital. Their special needs are often greater than hospital personnel can be expected to provide. Your presence or that of someone your family member knows will help things go more smoothly, but it does mean that you will have to spend a lot of time at the hospital or arrange to have a team of helpers do so.

You should make alternative arrangements, in advance if possible, when you will not be able to care for your family member in the hospital. Find out whether others in the family or friends are willing to give some of their time. It is perfectly okay to do this. No single person can do all the caregiving—you will need backup.

It is useful to know in advance how to hire a professional caregiver for some or all of the hospital stay. Once your family member is admitted, discuss any arrangements you are considering with the staff, which has experience and information that can be of help. (See Chapter 16 for more on hiring help in the hospital.)

◆   ◆   ◆

A fall brought Mr. R to the nearest hospital emergency room in the company of his home health aide. When his daughter arrived, she was told he had broken his leg and surgery would be required.

"I immediately felt overwhelmed because I knew that if this were the case, I would want to transfer my father to the hospital where his doctor practiced," she recalled. "The trouble was, I had no idea how to actually do this."

Much to her distress, she discovered that it can be difficult to transfer from one hospital emergency room to another, and that her only choice was to sign her father out against medical advice and to hire a private ambulance, which Medicare would not cover. "This plan sounded scary, and the last thing I wanted was to take my father into a potentially chaotic emergency room and start all over again." Still, she decided it was really important to have him in a hospital where his own doctor could take care of him.

Six hours after Mr. R had arrived at hospital number one, and dozens of phone calls had been made, he and his daughter were in an ambulance on the way to hospital number two. "I was a nervous wreck, but fortunately my father was not upset. He had no idea where he was or where he had been. In a sad way, the dementia was a protection."

Mr. R's daughter learned a lot from the experience. Getting your family member to the hospital of your choice takes advance planning. "I should have made sure his aide knew the hospital we wanted. Although I finally worked out the transfer, it was an expensive and time-consuming process that could have been avoided."

♦   ♦   ♦

WHAT SHOULD YOU ASK YOUR RELATIVE'S DOCTOR IN ADVANCE?

Your family member's doctor is the best person to ask about how to handle both emergency and planned hospitalizations. Try to schedule a telephone or in-person appointment to discuss the issue before the need arises. Here are some questions to ask:

- At which hospital or hospitals does the doctor have admitting privileges?
- If he or she has admitting privileges at more than one hospital, is one better suited to the needs of a person with dementia?
- In an emergency, should you ask the ambulance driver to take your relative to a particular hospital?
- What should you do if your family member is taken to a hospital where the doctor does not practice?
- How can you reach the doctor in a hurry if your relative is in the emergency room?

WHAT SHOULD YOU KNOW ABOUT THE HOSPITAL?

Once you know which hospital the doctor would choose for your relative, take some time to get to know the place. Many hospitals have a patient services department or a patient representative who can arrange for a tour and give you information about the hospital. It will be very helpful to take such a tour. Knowing your way around will make you feel more confident when you are actually caring for a hospitalized person who is confused and ill. Your relative will probably be reassured if you appear to be comfortable because the surroundings are familiar to you.

♦　♦　♦

Once Mr. R and his daughter finally made it to the second hospital, they had to wait in the emergency room for a hospital bed. Mr. R's daughter hadn't had anything to eat for many hours. Fortunately, she had previously taken a tour of the hospital, was able to find the cafeteria without much difficulty, and didn't have to leave her father alone for more than a few minutes.

"I thought how difficult it would be to try to find my way in a strange hospital. There are either lots of confusing signs or no signs at all. I was such a nervous wreck that I never would have found my way if I hadn't been there before."

♦　♦　♦

Most hospitals have a patient representative whose job it is to answer questions and help solve problems related to the hospitalization. Do not hesitate to ask about anything you do not understand or think you may need, such as:

- What information will the hospital need besides your relative's Social Security and Medicare numbers and insurance plan?
- Can some of the admission process be accomplished ahead of time for non-emergency hospitalizations?
- Is there a comfortable room where a patient who gets upset easily can wait during the admission process?
- Will a wheelchair be available? Where can it be found?
- What equipment should you bring for your family member?

- Does the hospital make any special arrangements for patients with dementia?
- What are the visiting hours? Can they be extended for the family of a patient with special needs?
- Under what circumstances will the hospital allow a family member to sleep over?
- Does the admissions office have a pamphlet about hospital procedures and any regulations family caregivers need to know?

You may want to talk with friends, family, and anyone else you know who has had a recent experience in that particular hospital. But it is important to remember that each person has his or her own perspective and may not see things as you do.

WHAT WILL THE INSURANCE COMPANY REQUIRE?

Some private insurance carriers require advance notification about certain medical procedures and hospitalizations. Following their guidelines will reduce the chance of problems with reimbursement. In case of an emergency admission, notify the insurance company as soon as possible. Find out what your family member's insurance company requires and add that information to the crisis kit.

WHAT IF YOU ARE CARING FOR MORE THAN ONE DISABLED PERSON?

If you are the caregiver for more than one person, you have a more complex situation for which to plan. If one person has to go to the hospital, who will care for the other? In some cases, using temporary respite services at a nursing home may be a better solution than trying to keep the other person at home. Arrangements can be made for a short stay while the family takes care of the person who is in the hospital. Alternatively, other family members or friends may be able to cover for you, or you may have to hire an aide.

WHAT ELSE CAN YOU PLAN IN ADVANCE?

Have plans for someone to take over as many of your responsibilities as possible—care of pets, plants, etc.—if your relative has to go to the hospital. This will help you focus on the task at hand without additional worries and to make some spare time to take care of yourself.

Of course, you cannot think of everything in advance. There will always be the unexpected. But the more preparations you can make, the more confident you will feel in your ability to help your family member with Alzheimer's disease in a crisis.

♦ 9 ♦

What to Do in an Emergency

When you are caring for someone with Alzheimer's disease, the last thing you want to do is make an unnecessary trip to the emergency room, but you also do not want to neglect a potentially life-threatening situation. This chapter will help you identify emergencies and offer suggestions on what to do if one arises.

IN THIS CHAPTER

Is This an Emergency?

What If You Are Not There When an Emergency Occurs?

How Should Your Family Member Get to the Hospital?

What Should You Do While Waiting for the Ambulance?

What Should You Do When the Ambulance Arrives?

What Hospital Will the Ambulance Go To?

What Will Happen in the Ambulance?

IS THIS AN EMERGENCY?

When something goes wrong with a person who has Alzheimer's disease, especially if the two of you are alone, it is easy to panic. Your relative may be very upset or in pain and not able to tell you how seriously hurt he or she is or even where it hurts. It is up to you to decide what to do. Is this an emergency? Should you call the doctor or 911? Should you take your relative to a hospital emergency room in your own car or in a taxi?

The first thing to do is to try and contact your relative's primary care physician unless you are sure that it is an emergency. In that case call an ambulance. Unfortunately, people get sick, and accidents often happen at the most inconvenient times—like weekends or in the middle of the night, when you cannot talk to the doctor immediately, or when a doctor who does not know your relative is "covering" for the regular doctor. You may then have to make the decision yourself.

Some signs of an emergency that always need immediate medical attention are:

- Loss of consciousness or a marked change in mental state.
- Sudden severe chest pain.
- A fall that causes severe pain or inability to move.
- An accident that results in a blow to the head.
- Uncontrollable bleeding.
- High fever accompanied by confusion and delusions.
- Difficulty breathing.
- Repeated or forceful vomiting.
- Failure to urinate for more than twelve hours.
- Sudden slurring of speech, loss of vision or balance, extreme weakness.
- Violent or uncontrollable behavior.
- Swallowing a poisonous substance.

Do not be afraid to go to the emergency room if you think the person you are caring for is seriously ill, even if he or she has none of the symptoms on the list. Trust your instincts. Don't let the possibility of being wrong stop you.

◆   ◆   ◆

Mrs. B and her husband, who was in the moderate stage of AD, were hanging up a picture together. Mr. B was on a ladder, and Mrs. B was telling him where to hammer in the nail. He fell off the ladder and hit his head on the floor. Mrs. B wanted to take him to the hospital, but he insisted he was fine and refused to go. Since he seemed okay, Mrs. B gave in to him.

A few days later, a tremor developed in Mr. B's right hand, and he complained of a severe headache. He still insisted that he did not want to go to the hospital. It was only when he lost consciousness that Mrs. B called an ambulance.

A CT scan revealed a massive subdural hematoma—an injury to the head causing bleeding in the area between the skull and the brain, which can result in pressure on the brain. Fortunately, this does not necessarily cause permanent damage if it is detected and treated early enough.

The doctor explained to Mrs. B. that people with AD have a bigger space around their brains than other people, so the bleeding may not cause symptoms for several days. In addition, they may not accurately report symptoms or judge their seriousness. That is why it is important to take a person with AD to a doctor or hospital immediately if he or she falls or receives any blow to the head.

◆　　◆　　◆

WHAT IF YOU ARE NOT THERE WHEN AN EMERGENCY OCCURS?

Whoever is caring for your family member should have clear instructions about what to do in an emergency, but if your relative still spends a lot of time alone, try to find someone who knows him or her and can be available when needed. Give that person a key to the house or apartment and tell him or her about the crisis kit and where it can be found. Put all the important papers in the kit.

The phone number of your relative's primary care physician, the poison control center, a taxi or car service that can be called, and the name and location of the hospital to which you want your family member to be taken should all be posted near the telephone.

If you are not with your family member, there is a chance that he or she will be taken to a hospital other than the one you have chosen. You may accept this or decide to have your relative transferred. It will be worth your while to find out in advance what the laws are in your area regarding the transferring of patients from one hospital to another.

HOW SHOULD YOUR FAMILY MEMBER
GET TO THE HOSPITAL?

In an emergency, you should call 911, the police, or the fire department, whichever provides emergency medical service in your community, to send an ambulance. The service will be free if you abide by the regulations in your locality regarding which hospital your relative will be taken to.

Ambulance personnel are called *EMTs—emergency medical technicians.* Although not doctors, they are specially trained to deal with medical emergencies, assess the patient's condition, and perform certain emergency first-aid procedures. In addition, they can contact hospital personnel for instructions and bring the patient directly into the emergency room, speeding up the admission process.

It is generally not advisable to take a very sick or injured person to the hospital on your own, but you may want to follow the ambulance in your car if you are concerned about how you will get home and taxis are not available or are too expensive.

WHAT SHOULD YOU DO WHILE
WAITING FOR THE AMBULANCE?

It may take some time for an ambulance to get to your relative's home. If it is an apartment building, be sure the dispatcher knows which apartment to come to; and inform the doorman, if there is one, that an ambulance is expected.

Make your relative as comfortable as possible. It is best not to move a person who has fallen and may have a broken bone or an internal injury. You can, however, adjust the temperature in the room, cover your relative with a blanket if necessary, put music on or turn it off, depending on what you think will make him or her feel better.

If your family member can understand what you say, he or she will be comforted to know that help is on the way and that you will not leave him or her alone.

Since emergency situations are stressful, preparing yourself and your relative for the emergency room may be the most constructive way to use the time until the ambulance arrives. Here are some things you can do:

- If time permits, call your relative's primary care physician in case you were not able to reach him or her earlier.

- If you do not have a crisis kit, assemble insurance documents, advance directives, and the *Profile of the Person with Memory Impairment* if it is filled out (see Chapter 7). Include a list of your relative's medications.

- Slip a small notebook and a pen or pencil into your pocket or purse. Once you are at the hospital, you will be able to jot down names of doctors and other hospital personnel, procedures, questions and answers, and reminders to yourself and others.

- If you have a cellular phone, take it along. If not, have lots of change or a telephone card for using the public phone.

- Make sure you have your own wallet, with identification, credit card, and some cash for food, reading matter, other incidentals, and to pay for a taxi, which may be needed if your relative is able to go home instead of being admitted to the hospital.

- If your relative is not dressed, bring along a pair of shoes, clothes, and a coat to be worn home in case he or she is not admitted to the hospital. Be sure not to bring valuables, such as expensive watches, rings, and other jewelry; and do not plan to leave more than a few dollars with your family member. An inexpensive watch is okay if he or she generally wears one at home.

- Let someone else in your family or a friend know that you are taking your relative to the hospital and could use a helping hand.

WHAT SHOULD YOU DO
WHEN THE AMBULANCE ARRIVES?

When the ambulance arrives, tell the EMT that your relative has Alzheimer's disease. Most EMTs know that they should use a calm, slow, non-threatening approach, but if your relative is getting upset, you may suggest they do something that has calmed him or her in the past. The EMT will examine your relative and decide if it is necessary to go to the hospital. In some localities, however, anyone over a certain age will automatically be taken to the hospital if the EMS is called.

WHAT HOSPITAL WILL THE AMBULANCE GO TO?

In a rural area, the suburbs, or a small city, there may be only one hospital where all the local doctors practice. A large city, however, will have many hospitals to choose from. When the situation appears very serious, the EMTs will probably insist on going to the nearest one, but if you prefer a particular hospital, ask them if it is safe to bring your relative there. If he or she is stable and the ambulance service is not too busy, they may be willing to do so, although sometimes at an extra charge. When you know in advance that the hospital of your choice is outside the limits of the emergency medical service, keep the names and phone numbers of private ambulance companies posted near the telephone.

WHAT WILL HAPPEN IN THE AMBULANCE?

In the ambulance, EMS personnel will tell you where to sit. During the trip you will be asked about your relative's medical and medication history. It will be easier to answer if you have this information available in writing in the *Profile of the Person with Memory Impairment.*

If your relative is in the mild or moderate stage and not extremely ill or unconscious, he or she will be aware of what's happening, but, because of the dementia, may give the EMTs information that is not accurate. You will have to tread a fine line between respecting your family member's autonomy and insuring that medical personnel get the correct information on which to base a diagnosis.

Once you have communicated all vital information to the EMTs, it is best to leave things in their hands. Their job is to get the patient to the emergency room as quickly and safely as possible. Once you arrive at the ER, though, there will be much for you to do.

· 10 ·

In the Emergency Room

Hospital emergency rooms are not easy places for anyone to be in, and they are particularly difficult for someone who has Alzheimer's disease. They can be crowded, noisy, and chaotic. Still, you may one day find yourself in the ER with a seriously ill or injured family member who is also suffering from AD. This chapter will tell you what to expect so you can prepare yourself emotionally and practically for what lies ahead.

IN THIS CHAPTER

Why Do People Go to the Emergency Room?

What Will Happen in the Emergency Room?

What Is Your Role in the Emergency Room?

Will Your Family Member Be Admitted to the Hospital?

Will You Need Extra Support in the Emergency Room or Afterwards?

WHY DO PEOPLE GO TO THE EMERGENCY ROOM?

Many different kinds of care are provided in the emergency room. We generally associate ERs with heart attacks or accidents, but other serious and potentially life-threatening conditions are often diagnosed and treated there. For example, when the cause of a problem is not clear and could be serious, a primary care physician might tell a patient to go to the emergency room for the kind of extensive evaluation that cannot be done in a doctor's office. And of course there are those weekends and holidays when doctors are not available and the ER may be the only place to receive immediate medical attention.

WHAT WILL HAPPEN IN THE EMERGENCY ROOM?

If your family member was brought to the emergency room in an ambulance, the EMT will give the admitting nurse a report on his or her status, medical history, and medications. The doctor who examines your relative will probably also ask you about the medical history and current problem. You may feel that you are being asked the same questions over and over. Try not to let this upset you; instead, think of it as an opportunity to be sure that everything is accurate, and to repeat that your relative has Alzheimer's in addition to whatever else is wrong.

Along with questions about your relative's medical history, expect the admissions representative to ask you about health insurance. If you have a copy of the *Profile of the Person with Memory Impairment* with you, you will have at your fingertips all the information you need to answer the questions you will be asked.

Be sure to tell the person who is taking the medical history if the symptoms of dementia have suddenly gotten much worse. This may be a sign of delirium—a temporary but severe confusion which may indicate a life-threatening condition and always requires immediate medical attention. (See Chapter 1 for information about delirium.)

Much of what happens next depends on your relative's condition. He or she may be treated immediately or have to wait while others, whose conditions are more critical, are cared for. If the cause of your relative's problem cannot be determined right away, it may be necessary to do a series of tests. In that case you should prepare yourself for what may be many hours in the emergency room.

Try to stay with your family member all the time. A familiar face and voice may keep him or her from getting more confused and agitated through the examinations and long periods of waiting. If someone on the staff asks you to leave, explain as calmly but firmly as you can that your relative has Alzheimer's disease and it will be easier for everyone if you can stay with him or her. Keep in mind that there may be situations that require you to wait outside, especially if the ER is very crowded.

◆ ◆ ◆

Mrs. S absolutely never complained about pain, so when she could not get up from the couch because of pain in her side, her husband Sam was very concerned. Since it was too late at night to call their regular doctor, and Sam was afraid that trying to move her would make things worse, he called 911, and Mrs. S was taken to the hospital in an ambulance.

At the hospital, Mrs. S cried out whenever she was moved or touched, but she could not be given any pain medicine until she had been examined, and blood and other tests were completed to discover what was wrong. The doctor suspected that she had broken a rib so X-rays were ordered.

When ER personnel asked Mrs. S what had happened, Sam surprised them by answering for her, since he knew that because of her dementia she would not remember. He told them she had fallen two days earlier, which might have explained how her rib had broken, although he was puzzled by the fact that she had not seemed to be in any pain at the time. Mr. S tried his best to comfort his wife while they waited for the results of the tests.

When the X-ray confirmed that Mrs. S had indeed broken her rib, she was given some pain medication. The doctor told them that they could go home since nothing more needed to be done. They were told to contact their regular doctor for follow-up treatment. Because of her age, the doctor suggested that she get a bone scan at a later time to see if she had osteoporosis. Sam realized that his being there to speak for his wife enabled the doctors to give her the best care.

◆ ◆ ◆

Whether or not you are allowed to stay with your relative in the ER will be based on many factors, including the rules of the hospital, the way the staff members prefer to work, and how many other patients are waiting. If one of them requires emergency treatment involving equipment and personnel, for instance, and the staff wants to be able to move swiftly with as few obstacles as possible, or if your relative needs care that may frighten or distress you, you may be asked to wait in another area.

When you feel it is appropriate, though, do not hesitate to insist on staying with your relative, but always try to remain courteous, and let everyone know that you are the caregiver.

WHAT IS YOUR ROLE IN THE EMERGENCY ROOM?

Your main job is to speak for your family member when he or she cannot do so. In Chapter 17 we will discuss strategies for being an assertive and effective advocate for a hospitalized person with AD without making enemies. Here are some things you can start doing in the ER:

- Find out which nurse is responsible for your family member and how long his or her shift lasts. When the shift changes, introduce yourself to the new nurse, giving your name and that of your relative. Say that you are the caregiver, and repeat that your relative has Alzheimer's.

- A series of tests and diagnostic procedures may be needed to discover the cause of your relative's symptoms. These might include taking blood, X-rays, and an electrocardiogram (EKG). Ask what tests have been done and when the results are expected back. Make a note of these details, and if the results do not arrive within the expected time, ask a doctor or nurse to check on them.

- You may have to spend several hours or more in the ER. If your relative would normally take medication during this time, do not give him or her medicine from home. Instead tell a member of the medical staff what medication your relative usually takes and at what time. If the staff feels it is appropriate, the medicine will be provided. If it is not, try not to worry. There is generally more danger in over-medicating a patient than in missing a dose.

- If there is a chance that surgery will be needed, your family member will not be allowed to eat or drink. Once surgery has been ruled out, find out if you can feed your relative. Often snacks and juice are available if you ask for them.

- If your relative is in a very noisy or cramped spot, see if he or she can be moved to a quieter place. Explain that the noise and activity are frightening your relative and making care more difficult.

DEALING WITH CATHETERS AND DIAPERS IN THE EMERGENCY ROOM

One of the most normal events—the need to use the bathroom—can become a problem in the emergency room for a person with AD. Even if your relative is able to use the toilet independently at home, he or she may not be allowed to do so in the ER. It is not uncommon for a catheter to be inserted to collect urine so it can be measured and tested. Or it may be done for the convenience of the staff. It is more sanitary and easier to have a catheter in place than to try to explain to a person with dementia how to use a bedpan. Similarly, diapers may routinely be put on all elderly patients, even those who are not incontinent.

Your relative may not understand why he or she is not being allowed to get off the bed, how the catheter works, or why a diaper is being used. If he or she becomes anxious, what can you do?

- Ask the nurse or doctor if there is a medical need for your relative not to get up and use the toilet. Very often there is no specific reason; it is just a general precaution.
- Offer to accompany your relative to the bathroom yourself or ask if an aide can assist him or her.
- If your relative can understand, show him or her that the urine is flowing into the collection bag at the side of the bed.
- If your relative does not use a diaper at home, tell this to staff members. If they want to protect the bed and make any accidents easier to clean up, ask them to place a few extra absorbent pads under your relative.

> • When you have done the best you can to make your relative reasonably comfortable, try distracting him or her with a discussion, pictures, or anything you can come up with to change the subject.

◆   ◆   ◆

During the four hours that had elapsed since Mr. D and his son arrived at the emergency room, he had had nothing to eat or drink. That was a precaution in case he needed surgery, since his stomach would have to be empty for anesthesia to be safely administered. As the hours wore on, however, his son was becoming concerned that he had gone so long without food or even water. No one in the ER seemed to know if or when an operation would be necessary. Finally, he called the admitting doctor's office and found out from the secretary that no surgery had been scheduled for that day.

"That was my cue that I could get my father something to eat. But before I gave him anything, I let the nurse who was assigned to him know that I had cleared it with his admitting doctor. Each thing that I was able to do for him felt like a small triumph."

A person with dementia seems so vulnerable in the hospital, but especially in the emergency room, where staff can be running from crisis to crisis.

◆   ◆   ◆

WILL YOUR FAMILY MEMBER BE ADMITTED TO THE HOSPITAL?

When the doctor in charge of the emergency room has the results of all the tests, you will be informed of the diagnosis and recommendations for further care. If your relative is to be admitted to the hospital, and a bed is available, arrangements will be made for a transfer to the appropriate unit. Sometimes it will be necessary to wait in the emergency room for several hours or even a day or two before a bed becomes available.

If your family member is to be released, however, a discharge plan will be discussed with you. It will usually include instructions for immediate care at home, a referral back to your relative's regular doctor, and a prescription for medication, if it is needed. Be sure that you will be able to get the new medication in time for the next dose. If you think you cannot, ask the hospital to provide you with enough to tide you over until you can get the prescription filled.

The next step is to take your family member back home. This can be difficult if you have arrived by ambulance. Consider asking a friend or family member to come to the emergency room to help you. If your relative cannot travel by car or public transportation, an ambulance or ambulette (a specially equipped van) may be ordered. You will have to pay for this service if it is not covered by your relative's insurance.

There are times when you, the caregiver, may have something to say about whether or not your relative is admitted to the hospital. If you feel very strongly that being in the hospital will make things worse and you prefer to take your family member home, and his or her doctor is satisfied that this is a safe plan, the hospital will generally cooperate. On the other hand, the hospital may be prepared to release your family member, but you may feel unable to provide the necessary care at home. In this case, discuss your concerns with the doctor in charge of the case. If admission is not an option, ask to speak to a social worker, who may be able to help you develop alternative plans, arrange for home care, and advise you on how to get the supplies you will need to care for your relative at home.

WILL YOU NEED EXTRA SUPPORT IN THE EMERGENCY ROOM OR AFTERWARDS?

You may want support for your relative and yourself while you are in the emergency room. Patients may remain in the ER for many hours, sometimes even days, and you will need a break. You may want to go home to get additional supplies or to rest.

As soon as you know whether your family member will be admitted to the hospital or need more care at home than before, start to mobilize your troops. Either contact the people you have already made arrangements with or ask one of your team to make calls for you.

Once the emergency has passed, your relative may be able to return home. It may take a while for both of you to recover from the crisis and get back to your normal routine. At first your relative may appear more confused and anxious than before, but the chances are good that this will pass.

It is also possible, however, that a stay in the hospital will be necessary, involving more decisions for you. In the next chapter, we will look at how you can prepare your relative and yourself for a hospitalization, whether it is planned or unexpected.

· 11 ·

What to Do When Hospitalization Is Recommended

It is a near certainty that a person with Alzheimer's disease will need to go to the hospital at some point, either for an emergency or a planned admission. Depending on what is wrong, the hospital stay may be as short as overnight or for an indefinite period of time. Hospitalization may be recommended for observation and tests, treatment of an acute illness or infection, adjustment of medication, or for an operation.

There are many issues for caregivers to consider when a doctor recommends treatment in a hospital for a person with AD. Hospitalization is in itself a crisis because it upsets the familiar routines and schedules, something that is always difficult for people with AD to deal with. What can you do to prepare for the challenge ahead?

IN THIS CHAPTER

Is There an Alternative to Hospitalization?

Should You Follow the Doctor's Recommendations?

What Should You Ask the Doctor Before Your Relative Goes to the Hospital?

How Can You Prepare Your Family Member for a Hospital Stay?

How Can You Prepare Yourself for the Hospitalization?

IS THERE AN ALTERNATIVE TO HOSPITALIZATION?

There is no question that hospitals are difficult places for people with dementia. For that reason, it is a good idea to explore alternatives. In many situations it is possible to get needed care outside a hospital. For patients with AD, this is generally preferable. Outpatient care can be provided in a day surgery center, a same-day unit in a hospital, or in a doctor's office. Your decision may also be influenced by the guidelines of your relative's insurance company.

Some people, however, are so anxious or sensitive to pain or touch that it is better for them to be treated in a hospital, where there are more choices for pain management. You may also feel that it would be too frightening to take your relative back home immediately after a procedure. If your relative lives alone or with someone who is not qualified to care for him or her, a hospital stay may make more sense. Do not automatically rule out the idea of inpatient care, but do investigate what other options are available.

◆   ◆   ◆

Mrs. K noticed that her husband Jack, who was in the moderate stage of AD, had begun to walk more slowly. At first she thought this was another symptom of Alzheimer's and that she should just accept it as an inevitable change. Then one day, as she was helping Jack get dressed, she noticed a small bulge in his lower abdomen and asked him whether it hurt. He said, "No," as he almost always did when she asked him if something was wrong, but she wasn't sure she should believe him. Maybe it just didn't hurt at that moment, and he couldn't remember that it hurt when he walked. Since she had never noticed the bulge before, she took him to the doctor.

The doctor examined him and found a small hernia. He recommended surgery and told Mrs. K to speak to the nurse about scheduling the operation. Mrs. K asked him if it would be necessary to stay over in the hospital after the operation. He said that because of Jack's age and other medical problems it would be safest if he did, although in some cases a day surgery center would be adequate. While she knew that people with Alzheimer's often do not react well to anesthesia and to being in a strange place, Mrs. K was afraid to neglect her husband's condition. Reluctantly, she made arrangements with the nurse to have the surgery performed a few weeks later.

◆　◆　◆

SHOULD YOU FOLLOW THE DOCTOR'S RECOMMENDATIONS?

Your family member's doctor may recommend the kinds of tests or procedures that require hospitalization, but before you go along with such a recommendation, ask the doctor the following questions:

- What does the procedure or test involve? Can the doctor or the hospital give you any written information about it?
- Is the procedure or test absolutely necessary? What will it accomplish?
- What might happen if the procedure or test is postponed?
- What might happen if the procedure or test is not done at all?
- What are the risks of the procedure or test?
- What kind of anesthesia will be used, if any? What will be the effect of the anesthesia on a person with dementia?
- Can the procedure or test be done on an outpatient basis?
- Will there be a prolonged recovery period, and what additional care is likely to be required during that time?
- Will it be possible to follow the instructions for aftercare?
- Will the procedure improve your relative's quality of life?

◆　◆　◆

Mrs. K was worried about whether she should go through with her plan to have her husband's hernia operated on. She remembered that the husband of one of the women in her support group had a hernia and had not agreed to an operation. "If Sally's husband didn't need to have the procedure, maybe Jack won't either," she thought to herself. She called her friend for the name of the doctor she had gone to with her husband. Mrs. K was not sure that this doctor would make the same recommendation for her husband, but she thought it was worth a try.

She hesitated to get a second opinion because she didn't want to offend their doctor, who was a long-time friend of the family. "I pushed myself to get over that, because I wanted to spare Jack and myself the stress of a hospitalization if I could." The second doctor agreed that Jack had a small hernia, which could be treated surgically. However, since the hernia was small and didn't seem to be causing a lot of discomfort, he recommended that Jack try using an abdominal support and return in three months for a follow-up appointment. This watch-and-wait approach seemed like a very reasonable alternative, so Mrs. K decided to try it. Jack walked much better when he wore the support, and she was able to avoid surgery, at least for the time being. She was very glad she had not rushed ahead and followed the first doctor's advice.

◆   ◆   ◆

Do not hesitate to get a second opinion to help you understand your choices and the pros and cons of each one. In the case of Mrs. K it was easy to follow the advice of the second doctor. However, when the situation is more complicated or the illness potentially life threatening and two doctors disagree, it will be hard to decide whose advice to follow. Under these circumstances you may even seek a third and fourth opinion to satisfy yourself that you are doing the right thing. Some health insurers even require a second opinion before certain procedures can be approved.

You do not have to make the decision by yourself. If your relative can understand the choices at all, ask what he or she wants to do. You may also wish to include involved family members in the decision-making process.

WHAT SHOULD YOU ASK THE DOCTOR BEFORE YOUR RELATIVE GOES TO THE HOSPITAL?

If you have decided to go ahead with hospitalization, these are some of the questions to ask the doctor who has recommended it:

- How much will he or she be involved in your relative's care during the hospital stay?
- Will he or she coordinate your relative's care?
- Will he or she select or recommend other doctors?

- Will he or she visit your relative in the hospital?
- Will he or she inform the hospital that your relative has AD?
- Does the chosen hospital make any special arrangements for patients with dementia?
- If the admission is not an emergency, can routine tests be completed before your relative is admitted?
- What is the best way to take your relative to the hospital? Will an ambulance be necessary?
- How long does the doctor expect your family member to stay in the hospital?
- How long is the recovery period likely to be?
- Will there be any pain? For how long? How can it be relieved?
- Will additional care be needed at home after discharge?

For a planned hospitalization, most insurance companies require notification and approval ahead of time. Check that the necessary approval has been obtained before you go.

HOW CAN YOU PREPARE YOUR RELATIVE FOR A HOSPITAL STAY?

Shortly before leaving for the hospital, give your relative only as much information as you think he or she can understand. Don't lie, just simplify. For example, you might say, "We're going to the hospital to take care of what is hurting you."

You may catch yourself talking about the hospitalization with the doctor or someone else in front of your relative as if he or she were not there. Other people, including medical personnel, may also do so. Try not to let this happen.

People with dementia are still able to pick up on the tone of what is being said and will know that something important is happening. Unfortunately, they may misunderstand what they hear and become confused or unnecessarily frightened. You will undoubtedly have questions or a need to talk with health providers or friends to relieve your own concerns. Try to get this support for yourself out of earshot of your relative.

If your family member is still able to understand the importance of advance directives, they should be prepared before the hospitalization. Ideally, these directives will have been discussed and completed in a routine manner while your family member was well and not under pressure. If they have not been, try to fill one out now, but do your best not to give the impression that you are expecting something bad to happen. Simply explain that everyone does this nowadays before going to the hospital for any reason.

HOW CAN YOU PREPARE YOURSELF FOR THE HOSPITALIZATION?

In addition to taking care of all the practical arrangements, you may need to prepare yourself emotionally for the hospitalization of your family member. Sometimes memories of other experiences in the hospital with that person or someone else will come to mind. Or perhaps a long-forgotten experience of your own will suddenly feel like it happened yesterday. Maybe the timing is just awful, and you are angry and disappointed because you have had to cancel important plans. All these feelings are understandable. Do not berate yourself for having them. Caregivers need to have as much compassion for themselves as they do for their relative with AD.

Try not to take on the whole responsibility yourself. If you are a person who does not like to ask for help, this is an opportunity to overcome some of your reluctance. Involve other family members and friends. Ask for support a little bit at a time. One person might go with you when you take your relative to the hospital; another might stay with you during the procedure. Then, during the recovery period, when it may be difficult to keep your relative occupied, family members and friends can take turns visiting.

When a person with AD is in the hospital, the caregiver's responsibilities will change. Although you might think that having your family member under twenty-four-hour medical care will lighten your responsibilities, this may unfortunately not be the case. In the chapters that follow, we will look at what it means to care for a person with Alzheimer's who is in the hospital.

PART THREE

◆ ◆ ◆

In the Hospital

· 12 ·

The Effect of Hospitalization on a Person with Alzheimer's Disease

Hospitals are set up to provide treatment and care for people who are ill or injured. They have many rules and regulations that are designed to keep things running smoothly. For patients and their families, however, hospitals can feel impersonal, confusing, and frightening. This is especially true for people with Alzheimer's disease, since being in the hospital can bring on symptoms and behaviors that are more severe than those seen at home. They also have special needs beyond their immediate medical problems and beyond what hospitals can be expected to provide, which makes a hospitalization stressful for both patient and caregiver, whose role in the hospital will be discussed in the next chapter.

IN THIS CHAPTER

Why Is Being in the Hospital Especially Difficult for People with Alzheimer's Disease?

What Effect Does the Stage of Dementia Have on a Person's Behavior in the Hospital?

What Special Needs Do People with Alzheimer's Disease Have when They Are in the Hospital?

WHY IS BEING IN THE HOSPITAL ESPECIALLY DIFFICULT FOR PEOPLE WITH ALZHEIMER'S DISEASE?

People with Alzheimer's disease become easily upset by restrictions and changes in their living environment. With all its strange noises, people, and equipment, the hospital may make them even more confused and anxious. They will also be expected to adjust to a new schedule, disrupting their normal daily routine, and may not understand that they now need to ask for help with things they usually do on their own. Since it is hard for them to find their way around in a new place, something as simple as locating the bathroom and getting back to bed may make them feel frustrated and irritable. They may also not realize that they are ill or in the hospital, and may experience necessary painful treatments and examinations as being attacked or threatened. This may cause them to:

- Have greater difficulty thinking and remembering.
- Be unable to care for themselves the way they did at home.
- Be more irritable, angry, depressed, and uncooperative.

Fortunately, for many of them these changes are only temporary, and functioning will gradually improve once the person returns home.

◆　　◆　　◆

Mrs. F, a frail woman of eighty-two, was hospitalized with a broken hip. When her daughter Dorothy arrived for her daily visit, she asked the nurse how her mother's night had been. The nurse said, "Fine," in a somewhat unconvincing way. Dorothy then asked if her mother had received the medication she usually took for the symptoms of AD.

After saying nothing for a moment, the nurse shook her head. "No," she said, adding in a whisper, "She was violent." Dorothy felt mortified and ashamed. "I pictured my tiny mother being led away in handcuffs."

What actually happened began about eleven o'clock at night when Mrs. F had been awakened from sleep, transferred to a gurney, and taken down to be X-rayed without a familiar face or voice to comfort her. As far as the hospital staff was concerned, this was not an unusual circumstance, since it is common for hospital patients to be taken for procedures at odd

hours. It probably never occurred to anyone how frightening it was to
Mrs. F and how difficult it is for a person with AD to cope with fear.

Back in the room sometime later, Mrs. F refused to take her medication
and pushed the nurse's arm away, spilling the cup of water the nurse was
holding. Dorothy asked the nurse if she had expected her mother to seriously
harm her. "Not really, but you know how they can get," was the reply.

♦ ♦ ♦

Some people believe the myth that everyone with Alzheimer's gets violent. This expectation can lead them to label even a mildly aggressive act as violent. In fact, such behavior is quite rare. If it happens at all, it is usually in the moderate stage of the disease.

Sometimes when the situation is examined closely, it turns out that the hospital staff is unaware of the special needs of a person with Alzheimer's. Although it is common practice in hospitals to awaken patients to take medication, this can be enormously distressing for those with AD, who frequently get more agitated in the late afternoon and may be particularly upset late at night. To the hospital staff, their resulting behavior may look like "noncompliance" or even aggression. In fact, such patients have been stressed beyond their ability to cope and are merely trying to protect themselves any way they can.

WHAT EFFECT DOES THE STAGE OF DEMENTIA HAVE ON A PERSON'S BEHAVIOR IN THE HOSPITAL?

People with only mild dementia may initially appear not to have any cognitive problems at all. Not realizing they need to be reminded about special instructions and helped to follow them, the hospital staff may understandably not be prepared when a patient makes mistakes, becomes confused, or gets angry.

For example, a person with AD is told not to put weight on an injured foot, but does so anyway because he or she forgets or did not understand the instruction. This may appear to be willful disobedience when, in fact, it is understandable behavior for a person with AD under these circumstances. Because they are sick and in a strange place, people in the mild stage of AD may behave as if they were in a more severe stage while in the hospital.

In the moderate and moderately severe stages of AD, people are more confused, forgetful, and frightened of being without their caregiver than before. They need constant supervision and reassurance to cope with the demands of a strange setting like a hospital, and may:

- Be more likely to become aggressive, shout, or cry for no apparent reason.
- Sometimes see and hear things that are not there.
- Disturb and frighten other patients and staff.
- Pick at their bandages and pull out IV lines.
- Not know where they are, perhaps believe they are at home, and not understand why strange people are in the room.
- Find it very hard to cooperate with staff.

People in the severe stage require a great deal of time-consuming physical care, such as help eating. If they cannot move by themselves, they need to have range-of-motion exercises, in which their arms and legs are moved for them to prevent them from tightening to the point where they cannot be moved at all. They also need to be turned frequently to prevent bed sores.

◆   ◆   ◆

Alice M learned how much additional care her father needed shortly after he was admitted to the hospital. "At first, I thought I should leave every-thing to the staff. They are professionals and know about taking care of sick people. I didn't want to get in the way."

She began to worry, though, when she noticed that her father seemed more confused than he had been at home. "The staff always seemed to be very busy and just couldn't take the time with my dad that he needed. And of course he didn't remember what they told him, like 'Here is the call button,' or 'Don't touch the bandage.' I could see that they were getting annoyed, and he was too." Consequently, she started to speak up more, explained what her father needed, and began taking more care of him herself.

"Maybe I was foolish at first, but I guess you can't really know in advance how it is going to be when a person with Alzheimer's is sick and in a strange place. But now I know, you have to be there for them all the time."

WHAT SPECIAL NEEDS DO PEOPLE WITH ALZHEIMER'S DISEASE HAVE WHEN THEY ARE IN THE HOSPITAL?

Feeling safe and secure is a basic need of people with AD regardless of the stage of their disease. So are self-respect and a feeling of being in control. These do not change in the hospital, but are simply harder to meet than at home. It is therefore essential to remember the dignity, individuality, and essential humanity of your family member while you or others are attending to his or her physical needs.

Regardless of the stage of dementia, it is never appropriate to assume that a person is beyond awareness and cannot be comforted by a gentle touch and kind words. People with AD need a great deal of support to benefit from a hospital stay, and it is unrealistic to expect the overworked staff to provide all of it. Some of the attention to special needs must come from the family or hired helpers, but how you treat your relative may serve as a model for staff members and hired helpers alike.

The fact is that people with AD need a lot of help in the hospital, even if they can manage alone at home. The active involvement of one or more family members can make a big difference. The next chapter will explore what you can do to smooth the way.

◆ 13 ◆

An Introduction to Your Role As a Caregiver in the Hospital

When people you care about are so sick they need to be in the hospital, it is natural to worry about them. When someone you care about who has Alzheimer's is in the hospital, you will worry not only about him or her getting better, but also about the symptoms of the disease getting worse. It is a new environment for both of you. Learning how to help your family member means learning how to work within the structure and realities of the hospital.

If your family member is having surgery or is in intensive care, you will be visiting, making decisions, and supervising rather than providing hands-on care. Once the immediate danger is past, he or she will be transferred either to a regular hospital room or a step down unit, both of which are intended for patients who no longer need intensive care. At that point, you may take a more direct role in caring for your relative.

It is important to remember that hospitals are set up to provide acute care. Their task is to treat the immediate cause of the hospitalization. Although some hospitals have special floors or units for patients with dementia, most do not.

IN THIS CHAPTER

Why Should You Tell the Hospital Staff That Your Relative Has Dementia?

What Can You Do for Your Hospitalized Relative?

Can You Do It All Alone?

WHY SHOULD YOU TELL THE HOSPITAL STAFF THAT YOUR RELATIVE HAS DEMENTIA?

Alzheimer's affects every aspect of hospital care. It is up to you to alert the hospital staff to the special AD-related needs of your family member, and to meet some of those needs yourself.

◆　◆　◆

Henry O's mother was hospitalized for tests to discover the cause of unexplained pain she had been experiencing for several weeks. He was concerned that she would be upset by being away from home and by the many tests that might be needed for the doctors to arrive at a diagnosis. While he knew it was necessary for her to be in the hospital, he was afraid that the nurses, doctors, and other staff members who would be dealing with his mother might not be able to handle her angry outbursts, her inability to communicate clearly, and her moodiness—all due to her Alzheimer's disease. Would these people who did not know her as well as he, or feel about her as he did, be understanding in caring for his mother, who could be a very difficult patient.

After making sure that his mother was in bed and relatively calm, he went out into the corridor. "I had to prime myself to take on the next task. Approaching the nursing station, I waited for someone to look up and then asked her who would be taking care of my mother. A very sweet nurse responded and began recording my mother's medical history. I did my standard number, telling her that my mother had dementia and giving her all the necessary information, which by now I had repeated four or five times."

Henry was to repeat that information many more times over the course of his mother's hospital stay. Still, he realized, remaining calm and patient was the best way to accomplish his goal: to make sure that everyone caring for her was aware of the needs and limitations caused by her Alzheimer's disease.

◆   ◆   ◆

When your relative first gets to the hospital, staff members will be focusing on the serious medical problem that has caused the hospitalization. They may not know that your relative has dementia unless you tell them. Sometimes the medical problem can be diagnosed more quickly and treated more effectively if the doctors know that the confusion they are observing is not a new symptom, but part of AD. If you have filled out the *Profile of a Person with Memory Impairment* (which is explained in Chapter 7), this is a good time to use it.

WHAT CAN YOU DO FOR YOUR HOSPITALIZED RELATIVE?

Can you think of yourself as a translator, mediator, advocate, supervisor, administrator, executive, interior designer, companion, and best friend? As a caregiver for a person with AD, you will play all these roles when your family member is hospitalized, and be expected to:

- Help him or her tolerate all the necessary procedures.
- Let the staff know about situations you think will be difficult for your relative to manage.
- Ask the staff what might be alternative procedures or routines to accommodate your relative's special needs.

In addition, there is much you will have to do for a person with AD that other people can do for themselves. Your role will run the gamut from making major decisions about medical care to helping with day-to-day tasks and finding safe and interesting activities to pass the time while your relative is in the hospital. In Chapter 16, we will talk more about the kinds of special help your relative may need.

♦   ♦   ♦

When Mrs. B went to visit her husband in the hospital, the nurses reported how pleased they were with his progress. He had injured himself in a fall from a ladder and, according to the nurses, was resting comfortably in his bed. When she approached him, though, she immediately noticed a scowl on his face, which told her that he was in pain. She pointed to the wrist he had bruised when he fell off the ladder, and asked him if that was bothering him. He shook his head, "No." She then asked him if he had a headache, and he said, "Yes." Mrs. B was relieved that she had figured out what was hurting him, and realized that only she knew him well enough to interpret his facial expressions. She told the nurse that he had a headache, and the nurse made arrangements for the doctor to come in and examine him.

♦   ♦   ♦

Since your family member will not always be able to explain what he or she needs or feels, you may have to interpret what your relative is trying to say. You have known this person for a long time and probably understand his or her special words, actions, and ways of expressing him or herself; but remember to let him or her do the talking whenever possible.

Caregivers of people with AD worry about how to keep them from being frightened, how to comfort them, how to help them know where they are, and how to make sure that, in their confusion, they do not put themselves in danger. Because they need company and supervision virtually all the time they are in the hospital, this requires a major commitment of time and emotional resources.

You can insure that your relative gets what is needed by being in the room as much as possible and by providing some of the care yourself. For example, you (or another family member) can help by turning him or her in bed and doing range-of-motion exercises. Before doing any of these tasks, though, be sure to check with the hospital staff.

OTHER THINGS YOU CAN DO

Caregivers can do a great deal to increase their hospitalized relative's feeling of well-being and self-esteem, and keep them looking and feeling attractive. Days in the hospital are long and tedious, and there is often too much time with nothing to do. You could fill that time by giving your relative a manicure, massage, or haircut—the kinds of activities you may not have time for at home. Depending on your family member's condition, he or she may be able to give you a hand massage or do your nails. Letting your relative experience the satisfaction of being a caregiver to you may help you both feel better.

CAN YOU DO IT ALL ALONE?

Think about how much you can and want to participate in the care of your family member in the hospital. For example, is it important for you to feed your family member? Is it reasonable to expect a member of the staff to do it? Do you feel that someone should be in the room with your relative at night? Can you take this on? Are there other people who can take turns spending the night? Be realistic in your expectations of the staff and of yourself. You may feel you have to hire someone to help out. Talk this over with family as well as staff members to find out what will be allowed.

The fact is, you cannot always take care of your family member on your own. You need backup so you can take frequent breaks. That is why every caregiver has to develop a support system. Let your friends and family help with the caregiving. Hire additional help if you need it and can afford it. (See Chapter 16 for information about hiring extra help in the hospital.)

Spending so much time worrying about your relative that you stop thinking about yourself would be bad for everyone involved. In the next chapter we will look at some of the things you can do to take care of yourself during this time.

· 14 ·

Taking Care of Yourself

What about you? You are working so hard to make everything right for your relative that even when you are at home, you find yourself worrying about what more you can do. If, however, you do not look after yourself, you probably won't be able to continue taking care of your relative. You may even begin to feel neglected and resentful. Here are some of the ways to help yourself.

IN THIS CHAPTER

How Can You Pace Yourself?

What Can You Do to Make Yourself More Comfortable in the Hospital?

What Kind of Social Support Can You Look for in the Hospital?

What about All Those Feelings?

HOW CAN YOU PACE YOURSELF?

You cannot accomplish everything at once. It is vital to set priorities. Since what has to happen first is not always obvious, you may need to get help deciding where to begin. Make a list and try to rank items by degree of importance, urgency, and feasibility. Sometimes it helps to do a few quick and easy things first, even if they are less important, just to give yourself and your family member confidence. Three guidelines that may help you pace yourself are:

- Do not try to do everything yourself. Ask other family members to pitch in.

- Hire help.

- Take breaks. Try not to be at the hospital twenty-four hours a day.

WHAT CAN YOU DO TO MAKE YOURSELF MORE COMFORTABLE IN THE HOSPITAL?

At first everything will seem strange. You will not know where to find things or what is permitted. Take a little time to get familiar with the unit where your relative is being treated as well as the hospital as a whole. Note the following suggestions:

- Introduce yourself to the unit clerk and ask to be shown around.

- Ask where you can find supplies, such as an extra blanket or pillow.

- Ask if a cot or a reclining chair may be put in the room if you have to stay overnight.

- See if there is a pantry with juice and other snacks for patients, and whether there is a place you can keep something for yourself.

- Find out where you can relax. There may be special places, such as a sun room, library, garden, chapel, or lounge, where you can go, with or without your relative, to relax, read a magazine, or take a break from his or her room.

- Visit the cafeteria and library; find the gift shop and ATM. You will feel much more confident in the hospital when you know your way around.

WHAT KINDS OF SOCIAL SUPPORT CAN YOU LOOK FOR IN THE HOSPITAL?

Hospitals provide a range of support for families of patients. It may take some doing to search them out, but here are some possibilities:

- Attend caregiver support groups. Whether or not the group is specifically for caregivers of patients with dementia, it can be a source of information and companionship.

- Meet with the social worker if you are concerned about any aspect of your relative's care or need help for yourself.

- Consult with the pastoral care team. Clergy of many denominations are generally available to meet with family members and patients. They can add both a practical and spiritual perspective. Even someone who is not of your faith may sometimes be helpful.

◆　◆　◆

Ever since Sandy's mother had been diagnosed with AD, her friends, who noticed how stressed she was, had been telling her to join a caregiver support group. She had given them all a thousand reasons why she was not interested. "I don't join groups or talk about my personal problems with strangers."

But after her mother had been in the hospital for about ten days, she found herself walking down the corridor feeling overtired and very much alone, when she remembered seeing a notice near the elevator about a caregiver support group. She went back to read it and discovered that it was meeting later that night. "I guess I was feeling so down that I decided to go," she said. "I figured that being in a group couldn't be any worse than feeling so alone."

Sandy was surprised at how comforting it was to be with people who completely understood what she was going through. She also got some helpful tips about taking care of her mother, and decided to go again the following week, even if her mother had already been discharged from the hospital. "I realized that I could be more help to my mother if I got some help myself."

WHAT ABOUT ALL THOSE FEELINGS?

You may be subject to as many ups and downs as your relative during the hospitalization, feeling hopeful one day and discouraged the next, grateful to the staff at times and furious at other times. This is natural, but it does add to your stress. People with dementia may be particularly vulnerable in the hospital, but they can also show remarkable resilience and wisdom. There are times when your relative may not be as distressed as you are.

- Try not to overreact when there seems to be a setback in your relative's condition. The course of a hospitalization is not necessarily straight or even. Of course, if you think his or her therapy should be different or if you have other concerns, speak to the doctor or appropriate staff member. Refer to the Appendix to determine who is the best person to talk to.

- Try to keep your sense of humor. Finding the humor in a painful, difficult, or frustrating situation may reduce your stress, ease your pain, and perhaps even help you come up with the solution to a difficult problem.

- Be realistic. You cannot cover all bases or control all the different forces that affect the outcome of a hospitalization. Remember that you are only human and are doing the best you can—which is good enough.

- Keep in mind that caregiving is not your only responsibility. Do not sacrifice your job or relationships with other family members and friends. Caregiving may play a central role in your life right now, but it is important to maintain and enjoy your other relationships as well.

◆   ◆   ◆

Sylvia is the first to admit that as much as she loves her father and wants to be sure he gets the best care in the hospital, there are days she feels that she has reached the end of her rope.

"One day when I came to visit my dad and he asked me, 'When am I going home?' for the tenth time, I felt that I just couldn't bear to hear it

anymore. I needed to take a break. As pleasantly as I could, I told him that I had an important business meeting. Then I went around the corner to the movies, bought popcorn and soda, put everything else out of my mind, and enjoyed the show. When I went back to the hospital a few hours later, I was entirely ready for my father's inevitable questions, and answered as sweetly as I could every time he asked."

◆   ◆   ◆

Do not underestimate the value of taking care of yourself. Since people with dementia often do not realize how hard you are working and rarely, if ever, express their gratitude, you will have to take responsibility for your own well-being in addition to that of your family member.

· 15 ·

Decisions

When a person with Alzheimer's disease is hospitalized, family caregivers may be faced with especially difficult questions about how to make sure he or she receives the most appropriate care. The family decision maker will have to consider the seriousness of the illness or condition that has caused the hospitalization, as well as the stage of AD and state of health in general.

In the final analysis, maintaining or improving the person's quality of life may be more important than treating or curing an illness. When the severe stage of dementia is reached, it may be necessary to make a decision about whether to continue aggressive treatment and life-prolonging measures or whether it would be better to chose palliative care.

IN THIS CHAPTER

Who Makes Decisions for a Person with Alzheimer's Disease?

What Kinds of Decisions Can You Expect to Make?

Who Can Help You Make Decisions?

Should You Approve a Particular Procedure?

Should You Ask for a Second Opinion?

WHO MAKES DECISIONS FOR A PERSON WITH ALZHEIMER'S DISEASE?

In the early stages of the illness it will be more difficult to determine your relative's competence. If there is any question, either his or her physician or a psychiatrist should be asked to make an evaluation. At some point, however, the dementia caused by Alzheimer's disease will become so severe that your relative will clearly no longer be capable of making medical care decisions and someone else must act on his or her behalf.

For the purposes of this discussion, we are assuming that your are that person. Ideally, you and your relative will have already taken the steps described in Chapter 6—you have been designated as the decision maker, and your relative has made his or her wishes about medical care known. If this has not already been done, and you are the patient's closest family member, the medical staff will generally turn to you to make decisions. (The spouse is considered the closest relative, followed by an adult child.)

DEFINITIONS

Competence: Competence to consent to medical treatment involves being aware of the condition for which the treatment is being offered, the probable effects of the treatment, and the consequence of refusing it.

Guardianship: When a person becomes incapacitated and has not made any provisions in advance for taking care of his or her medical or other affairs, it may be necessary to have a legal procedure in which the court declares that person incompetent and appoints someone—a guardian—to manage financial affairs and make medical care decisions.

If there is serious disagreement about a decision among family members, or the family and the doctor, and there is no advanced directive, it may be necessary, as a last resort, to have a legal proceeding in which the court will appoint someone (it could be you) to be your relative's guardian.

Advance directives will provide insight into your relative's values and intentions, and help you make the many decisions with which you will be faced. If they have not been prepared, then your decisions should be based on what you believe are his or her best interests. Always remember that your job is to make the decision you think expresses your family member's point of view, even if it differs from your own. This will not always be easy, and in the case of end-of-life decisions, it may be extremely difficult to act even when you are following the guidelines your relative has provided.

◆　◆　◆

When Howard, a ninety-two-year-old man with moderate stage Alzheimer's and severe heart disease, refused to eat, drink, or take his medication, his family begged him to change his mind. The doctor said Howard could be kept alive if he were fed through a feeding tube inserted into his stomach.

Even though his advance directive clearly stated that he did not want this intervention, his daughter Julie insisted that it be given a chance. "I'm sure Dad would change his mind if he realized how much he means to us." Howard's wife and son, on the other hand, believed that Howard's wishes should be respected and were finally able to convince Julie. Because those wishes had been clearly stated, his family could take comfort that it was fulfilling them, and a possible disagreement about his care was avoided.

Guided by his advance directive, Howard's family enrolled him in a hospice program, which kept him comfortable and gave him pain medication, but did not attempt to prolong his life with a feeding tube or other extreme measures. The hospice also encouraged Howard's family members to be at his bedside and hold his hand, and provided comfort to them in their grief. "Dad's death seemed peaceful and pain free," Julie said. The hospice helped him die the way he wanted to, and helped my family get through this really difficult experience together."

◆　◆　◆

WHAT KINDS OF DECISIONS CAN YOU EXPECT TO MAKE?

You will be asked to make many decisions about your family member's care while in the hospital. They will range from day-to-day matters such as room arrangements and approval for treatments and procedures to wrenching end-of-life issues. The more severe your relative's dementia is, of course, the more decisions you will need to make on his or her behalf.

Many of these will have to do with very personal feelings, values, and religious beliefs; and may involve continuing treatments to prolong life, but at a level you do not consider worthwhile. For example, when your relative has not made his or her wishes known, you may have to decide whether or not to use a feeding tube if he or she is no longer able to swallow, mechanical ventilation to assist breathing, and medications that may relieve pain but possibly shorten life. One of the first decisions you will be asked to make when your relative is admitted to the hospital is whether to sign a *do not resuscitate (DNR)* or *do not intubate (DNI)* order. This can be very upsetting, especially if you do not understand its purpose.

WHAT IS A DNR?

A do not resuscitate order tells the staff that **only if a patient's breathing or heartbeat stops,** no effort should be made to restore it. This includes mouth-to-mouth resuscitation, CPR, insertion of a tube to open the airway, external chest compression, electric shock, open-chest massage, and injection of medication into the heart to try to restart it.

If a DNR is not signed, then hospital personnel are obligated to do everything possible to save the patient's life. It is important to understand, however, that the DNR order is **only about resuscitation** and will not prevent a patient from receiving other kinds of treatment. Even when a DNR has been signed, all efforts will be continued to keep a patient comfortable. You can cancel a DNR at any time and sign another one if circumstances change. The idea behind the DNR is to avoid putting a person through the experience of being resuscitated if he or she will probably have a very poor quality of life afterwards due to significant brain damage, irreversible coma, or other severe impairments.

If you are the designated decision maker for a person who cannot sign the DNR order, you may be asked to do so when:

- Your relative has a terminal condition with the imminent expectation of death.
- Your relative is permanently unconscious.
- Resuscitation would be medically useless or involve risks of serious impairment.

Note: A reference to a DNI, which stands for *do not intubate,* may be included as part of the DNR form. This procedure, which involves passing a tube connected to a ventilator into the body, is sometimes necessary to restore breathing. After intubation, the patient may permanently need to be on a ventilator to breathe. Unless permission to withdraw this support was explicitly given by the patient in an advance directive, the person may be forced to remain on a ventilator indefinitely, after all hope of recovery is lost.

WHO CAN HELP YOU MAKE DECISIONS?

Since making these decisions is an awesome responsibility, try to get as much information as you need in each situation. You might find it helpful to talk to your relative's doctor and any specialists who are involved, in addition to a social worker at the hospital. Be prepared to ask questions and write down all the answers you get.

Once you have gathered the necessary information, involve everyone who can help you decide. This may include physicians, nurses, social workers and hospital chaplains, as well as spiritual advisors outside the hospital, friends, family, and even your relative, if he or she is able to participate. Under these very difficult circumstances, it is important to get as much support as you can and to share this responsibility.

Once you have made the decision, try not to undermine yourself with doubts and second guesses. You can, of course, learn from the experience and bring any new information to the next decision you are faced with.

✦   ✦   ✦

Mr. V was hospitalized because his lungs had filled with fluid. He had also been complaining that his back hurt. After about a week in the hospital, his breathing was much better, and the doctor suggested that, while he was there, he have a myelogram to determine the cause of his back pain. It would involve injecting dye into his spine and then viewing it with an X-ray-like device.

As Mrs. V told it, "He seemed to be agreeable to the plan, but when he was wheeled into the room where the procedure was to take place, he absolutely refused to sign the consent form. He kept trying to get off the examination table, and became irritable and angry. He wouldn't let anyone touch him. There was clearly no way to convince him to go through with it, and I just didn't feel right telling the technician to go ahead against his will. I think he refused because he didn't understand what was going on and got frightened."

In this particular case, there was no danger in going along with his wishes. Fortunately, Mr. V's back pain got better without treatment. Mrs. V learned from the experience that she could no longer leave medical decisions to him. "Having to decide for him is a heavy responsibility. I wish we had talked more when he was still able to think clearly about the kind of care he would want."

✦   ✦   ✦

SHOULD YOU APPROVE A PARTICULAR PROCEDURE?

You may be asked to make decisions about diagnostic or treatment procedures. Before giving or withholding approval, it is important to know what the risks and benefits are likely to be. For example, a quadruple bypass operation on a man in the moderately severe stage of dementia may make his dementia more severe and not improve his quality of life enough to justify putting him through the trauma of the surgery. Here are some questions, not unlike those to be asked about procedures before hospitalization, that may help you make the decision:

- What is the aim of the procedure or treatment?
- What, if anything, will be learned from the procedure?
- How will that information be used?

- Will it improve your family member's quality of life?
- Will it improve your family member's chances of recovery?
- What are the risks of the procedure or treatment?
- What are the consequences of not doing the procedure or treatment?
- What alternative treatments are available?

These questions will help you decide if your relative is likely to get "too much" medical treatment. What should you do if you think he or she might not be getting enough? You may be worried, for example, that certain tests or treatments are not being done. Ask why. Does it have to do with your relative's age, medical condition, stage of dementia, or the cost of the test? These may or may not be valid reasons for omitting what may be a useful procedure or treatment.

◆　◆　◆

After Mrs. H's hip operation, a catheter was inserted because she was not supposed to get out of bed or even use a bed pan for a while after the surgery. A few days later the catheter was removed with the expectation that she would urinate on her own within twelve hours.

Late that night, when she did not urinate within the expected time, an attempt was made to reinsert the catheter. Mrs. H fought against this confusing intrusion. The head nurse called her daughter to say that Mrs. H was not cooperating and that a serious medical problem might develop if she did not urinate before the twelve hours were up.

"I told her that by my calculations it was only eleven hours. 'Why not wait a little longer, and I will come back to the hospital,' Mrs. H's daughter suggested. Fortunately she lived nearby." "I took a taxi, and by the time I raced in, my frantic mother had wet herself. Far from being upset, I was glad she had been spared an unnecessary procedure. I sang my mother to sleep and walked home, relieved but completely exhausted."

◆　◆　◆

SHOULD YOU ASK FOR A SECOND OPINION?

The fact that a person has AD adds to the complexity of the medical decision-making process. There are times when you or your relative may want another opinion about how to proceed. Most doctors understand how difficult it is for someone in your position to make these decisions, and will respect your desire to seek additional information. Even though you may feel uncomfortable about asking for a consultation with another physician, it is your right to do so.

Asking for a second opinion does not necessarily mean you are dissatisfied, only that you are seeking as much information as possible to make an informed decision. You may want to talk to a physician who you believe is more knowledgeable about Alzheimer's or another aspect of medical care, or you may feel more comfortable asking the doctor to do so for you.

It is often difficult to change physicians in the hospital because it creates a potentially awkward situation among colleagues. Try, if you can, to find a way to work with the doctor who has been assigned to your relative. If that is not possible, ask this doctor to have a consultation with an expert on the issue in question.

As the caregiver and medical decision maker of a person with AD, you have to be assertive yet diplomatic when dealing with physicians and hospital staff, patient and caring when dealing with your relative, and knowledgeable about both AD and the other medical problem or problems your family member has. It is a heavy burden, but one you do not have to shoulder on your own. The key is to find allies to help you seek out information and weigh the pros and cons of every decision you must face.

· 16 ·

Supervising Your Family Member in the Hospital

If you have been responsible for the care of a person with Alzheimer's disease, you might think of a hospitalization as a respite from your daily duties. Quite the contrary is true. You will probably find yourself spending more time than usual with your relative and in a place where your choices about what to do and how to do it are more limited. Anything you can do to help your family member feel comfortable and secure will make the hospital stay more bearable for both of you, and may even help recovery go faster.

IN THIS CHAPTER

What Kind of Special Help Does Your Family Member Need?

How Much Supervision Does Your Family Member Need?

How Can You Arrange for Enough Help in the Hospital?

How Do You Go about Hiring Help?

WHAT KIND OF SPECIAL HELP
DOES YOUR FAMILY MEMBER NEED?

People with AD need help with what may seem simple and ordinary to others:

- They may not know how or remember to use the call button and may need someone to push it for them.

- They may not understand hospital rules, may go places and touch things they should not, and could use a person to distract them with a safe activity.

- They may not realize that the IV in their arm is attached to a pole that must be taken along with them when they get out of bed. Someone needs to push the pole for them and make sure they do not leave it behind or hurt themselves with it.

- They may not be able to find the bathroom or remember to call for help if they need assistance getting there; or they may get off the toilet by themselves because they usually do at home, not understanding that they are now too weak to manage without help. Someone should accompany them to prevent them from falling and help them if they are no longer capable of using the toilet on their own.

- They may not remember the instructions they are given—for example, to refuse foods they are not supposed to eat or to stay in bed when their treatment plan calls for complete bed rest—and need someone to remind them repeatedly.

- They may fall while trying to climb over the side rails, which are intended to keep them safely in bed. Reminding, comforting, and distracting are the best strategies for avoiding physical or chemical restraints.

- They may not understand how to fill out the menu, or be able or want to eat the food that is brought to them. They may need someone to help them make appropriate food choices or choose for them. They may require help eating or need to be fed.

DEFINITIONS

Chemical restraint: A drug given to control pacing, restlessness, and uncooperative behavior.

Physical restraint: Any device which limits a person's ability to move freely. Examples are hand mitts, soft ties or vests, leg and arm restraints, wheelchair bars, and geriatric chairs.

Geriatric chair: A very stable, well-balanced chair with a high back and a tray in front attached to its arms to prevent the person from getting up on his or her own.

If your relative is able to get up and walk around, there is a risk that he or she will wander away and get lost. Patients with AD have been known to leave the hospital floor or go into a maintenance closet, linen chute, or other dangerous place. The best way to guard against this is to be sure your family member is supervised around the clock. If you or someone else cannot be there all the time, try to get your relative assigned to a room that requires him or her to pass the nursing station before reaching an exit. If this means a room change, your relative's doctor is the best person to make sure it happens.

◆   ◆   ◆

Susan's husband David, who was in the mild stage of AD, had been taken to the hospital with terrible abdominal pain. Tests revealed that he had gallstones. He was told that if he did not eat certain foods, including ice cream, he would not need an operation. There was another patient in the hospital room whose family always brought him treats. When Susan arrived one day, she found David happily eating some ice cream his roommate's family had given him. She realized that unless she stayed with him all the time, she would have to put a sign where other people could read it, saying, "David is on a special diet. Check with the nurse before offering him any food."

◆   ◆   ◆

HOW MUCH SUPERVISION DOES
YOUR FAMILY MEMBER NEED?

In general, it is better to have too much supervision and companionship for your family member than too little. The aim is to prevent a problem rather than to wait until it happens. If your relative becomes agitated, noisy, or cannot sleep at night, he or she may be given medication that is supposed to have a calming effect. It may, however, cause a person with dementia to become more confused and, in some cases, more agitated. If you, another family member, or a hired companion is there, it may be possible to calm or distract your relative without the use of restraints or medication to control behavior.

Physical restraints can make people angry and frightened, even causing them to injure themselves while struggling to break free. Sometimes seating a patient in a geriatric chair (called a *geri chair* for short) will keep him or her securely contained without feeling tied down. There are times when, for the patient's own safety, physical restraints are the best alternative. Again, adequate supervision by someone who understands his or her needs may make it possible to avoid them.

Once you have decided how much supervision your family member needs, you will have to figure out what combination of family, friends, and hired help will cover all the bases.

HOW CAN YOU ARRANGE FOR ENOUGH HELP
IN THE HOSPITAL?

Ideally, family members and friends will visit, but they may not come on their own or at the times you need them most. Ask for their support, and work with them to schedule visits in a way that will be truly helpful to you. These visitors may not know how to care for your relative themselves, but at least they will know how to ask for help. When your relative has other visitors, you might use the time to meet with a staff member or take a break and do something for yourself.

Sometimes, however, even family and friends cannot provide all the care and supervision needed, and it will be necessary to hire help. You may find that you and your friends and relatives will be available during the day and in the early evening hours. It is during the night, however, that people with AD often need the most support—more support, in fact, than can realistically be met by the hospital's night staff.

If no one among family and friends is able to stay overnight, it will be necessary to hire help for these hours, especially if your relative has been staying awake and needs constant reassurance or has to go to the bathroom frequently.

◆　　◆　　◆

When Mrs. T was admitted to the hospital with heart palpitations, her husband was afraid that being alone in a strange place would make things even worse for her. The admitting clerk suggested that he hire a companion to stay the night with Mrs. T, allowing Mr. T to go home and get some rest after spending his days at the hospital. He welcomed the idea and was glad to know that a companion could be hired through the hospital, which meant having a person who would be familiar with hospital routine and even some of the staff.

"When the companion arrived, I told her about my wife and gave her a list of the important people in her life and how they were related to her. I wanted her to be able to talk to my wife and to recognize the names she mentioned. I also stressed that I could be called at any time of the night." The companion had worked with Alzheimer's patients before and knew just what to expect.

"By the time I left, I felt calm and satisfied that I had done a pretty good job so far. Even my wife, who had been in a terrible state when we first arrived, seemed strangely contented. She thought she was in a hotel and was pleased with the service. I did not contradict her, but went home to get some much needed sleep."

◆　　◆　　◆

HOW DO YOU GO ABOUT HIRING HELP?

The best person to hire is someone who meets your relative's needs and whom you can afford. Possibilities include:

- **Paid companions**, who will keep your relative company.
- **Aides,** who will wash, feed, and take your relative to the bathroom.
- **Licensed practical nurses (LPNs),** who can take blood pressure and temperature readings and may administer medications except for narcotics.
- **Registered nurses (RNs),** who can provide full nursing care

Hospitals often have a private duty nurse office to help you hire companions, aides, or nurses. These professionals are usually quite expensive, but have the advantage of being familiar with the hospital. The cost, of course, will increase with the level of expertise. If you want to bring in someone who was taking care of your relative at home or from an outside agency, check with the head nurse or nurse manager about hospital rules and procedures. You may be referred to the department that reviews the credentials and insurance of companions who are not on staff.

Do not have your hired helper do things he or she is not authorized to do. Also, check with the agency or hospital office to be sure you are hiring someone whose skills and job definition fit the needs of your family member.

The informal network is often a good source of information about hiring help. Ask other family caregivers how they have found people to care for their relatives in the hospital. Many hospitals have people on staff called *patient representatives*, who can help you negotiate the hospital system and make arrangements for your family member's special care needs.

WORKING WITH YOUR HIRED HELPER

Unfortunately, your work is not over after you have hired extra help. It is important to tell the person you have hired about your relative's needs and preferences, and what you expect him or her to do.

Plan to talk with your helper periodically, in person or on the telephone during the day, and in the morning, if he or she has been with your family member at night. Ask specific questions in order to get useful information. If you ask, "How are things?" or "How did everything go?" you will generally be told, "Fine." Instead ask, "Was my relative in pain?" "Was he nauseous?" "What medications was she given?" "Was he agitated?" "How many hours did she sleep?" "How many times did he go to the bathroom?"

Do not expect a hired person to show the same warmth and devotion to your family member as you do, but expect this person to behave in a professional manner when caring for your relative. If the first person you hire does not seem to be relating well to your relative, try to find someone else about whom you feel more confident.

Even when you hire private help, the hospital always has the ultimate responsibility for the patient's well-being, so do not neglect your relationship with the staff. In the next chapter we will look at how you can work most effectively with staff members.

· 17 ·

Working with the Hospital Staff

The people who work in the hospital have become comfortable there. They know their way around and how to find what they are looking for. You, on the other hand, may feel extremely vulnerable in these new surroundings even though you generally feel confident and self-assured in your own home or office. Nevertheless, their goal is the same as yours—to provide the best care possible. It is therefore best to work together.

Establishing and maintaining a good working relationship is a two-way street, but you may have to take the initiative. If you approach staff members with a positive attitude and assume good will on their part, things are more likely to go well.

IN THIS CHAPTER

What Is the Best Way to Build a Relationship with the Hospital Staff?

What Will the Hospital Staff Expect from You?

How Can You Communicate Effectively with the Hospital Staff?

How Can You Help the Hospital Staff Understand and Care for Your Family Member?

Who Can Help if You Have a Problem?

WHAT IS THE BEST WAY TO BUILD A RELATIONSHIP WITH THE HOSPITAL STAFF?

When your family member is in the hospital, you will be relying on the medical expertise of the staff to help him or her get well. Staff members, in turn, will rely on you for information and help that only a family member can provide. When staff and family work together, the patient is most likely to get the best care, minimizing stress and distress for all concerned.

Once your relative is in a hospital room, you should arrange a meeting with the nurse who is in charge of the unit and coordinates patient care. While discussing your relative's special needs would be a good time to give him or her a copy of the *Profile of the Person with Memory Impairment* and to express any anxieties or concerns that you might have about the hospitalization.

If you would like to take part in your relative's care, let the nurse in charge know that you can be available when needed. Find out whether it is reasonable to expect that the staff will do what is normally done for your relative at home.

Asking about the routines and regulations and the roles of the staff members caring for your relative will help you know the kinds of questions you can ask, and what to tell each of them about your relative. It also shows that you are eager to work with the staff in a constructive way.

WHAT WILL THE HOSPITAL STAFF EXPECT FROM YOU?

The first thing the staff will probably do is ask you for information about your family member's medical history and what has brought about the hospitalization. Even if you have given this information in the emergency room or to the admissions clerk, use this opportunity to begin to develop a relationship with the staff.

Most staff members will give you the feeling that they are glad you want to be involved in caring for their patient. Some may be less welcoming or may seem to be ignoring you. Try not to get angry. They may be under enormous pressures that are not obvious to you. It will be more productive to try to initiate positive interactions with them.

♦   ♦   ♦

By the time Mr. Z had been in the hospital for several weeks, his wife had come to know the aides who generally worked on the unit. Many had developed an easy way of chatting with Mr. Z, who enjoyed talking with them. "One aide, however, seemed to get pleasure out of getting my husband to carry on, raise his voice, and say inappropriate things. I noticed that visitors and other staff would sometimes watch these events and smirk, but I never saw anyone tell the aide to stop. It looked like I would have to do something."

At first, Mrs. Z distracted her husband and moved him away from the aide when she saw it was about to happen again. "After a while I decided that the aide might not know how much it upset me that she was behaving this way with my husband. I told her that it made me feel terribly embarrassed and sad to see my husband so out of control."

Mrs. Z's approach was effective because it did not blame or accuse the aide, but brought the matter to her attention in a way she could accept.

♦   ♦   ♦

HOW CAN YOU COMMUNICATE EFFECTIVELY WITH THE HOSPITAL STAFF?

Successful communication is a skill worth practicing when your relative with AD is in the hospital. Here are some strategies to ease the way:

- *Pick your time carefully.* When you approach a staff member, find out if this is a good time to speak with him or her. If not, ask when it would be more convenient.
- *Prepare what you want to say ahead of time.* Even though you think you know exactly what you want to say, it is best to write down your questions or concerns in advance.
- *Approach the staff with a positive attitude.* At times you may feel overwhelmed, embarrassed, frustrated, or just tired, but try to bring a positive attitude to your interactions with all staff members. If you can remain calm, pleasant, and friendly, staff members will probably do the same.

- *Acknowledge the staff's needs and priorities.* Preface your requests and questions with phrases like, "I know how busy you are," "I realize how difficult my relative is," and "I appreciate how much extra time you are giving my relative."

- *Offer suggestions in a constructive way.* If you notice that the staff is having difficulty with your relative—with feeding, for example—you might suggest something that has worked at home. Be aware, though, that hospital rules and restrictions may prevent staff members from always doing what you would like.

- *Be realistic.* Since providing special care for dementia patients is difficult and time consuming, try to ask only for changes that are absolutely necessary to your relative's well-being and care. Remember that you are asking a busy and hurried staff to slow down, spend more time with your family member, or come back at another time. You may be asking for something that is not normal procedure, such as accompanying a patient to tests. Explain that what you are asking for will make life easier for everyone. Volunteer to do the task yourself if a staff member cannot. But also be prepared to have your request turned down. You then can decide if the issue is worth pursuing, or if it is better to just let it go. Pick your battles carefully, and save getting angry as a last resort.

HOW CAN YOU HELP THE HOSPITAL STAFF UNDERSTAND AND CARE FOR YOUR FAMILY MEMBER?

Your relative is in the hospital because he or she needs the expert care of the medical staff. Unfortunately, there will be times when AD makes it impossible for your family member to understand or do what the staff asks. When this happens, some staff members may misunderstand and use the term *noncompliant.* They may think your relative is intentionally being uncooperative. Due to the pressure of time, they may get frustrated and cancel or postpone a procedure.

You can be helpful at such times because you have seen your relative behave like this before. The behavior management strategies that have worked for you in the past may also help the staff. Once staff members understand your relative's needs and manner of communicating, most of them will be able to get the cooperation they need. If you have filled out the *Profile of the Person with Alzheimer's Disease*, the staff may use the information in it when you are not available to provide explanations or advice about difficult behavior.

♦   ♦   ♦

Mrs. C had moderately severe Alzheimer's and was frequently ill-tempered with the hospital staff. Her son Jack was concerned, but also thought he could help.

"The nurses probably thought I was nutty, but when they told me Mom had been kicking up a fuss, I asked them if she had had a bowel movement that day. Past experience had taught me that when she was more irritable and difficult than usual, constipation was often the problem."

Jack told the nurse that he suspected Mrs. C was constipated, and suggested that she be given a glycerin suppository every evening, which is what he did at home. A suppository is not the same as a laxative, and it usually helps ease a bowel movement in a gentle way.

"Since I wanted so badly to help my mother, I was more than a little pleased when the nurse readily agreed. It's amazing what you have to learn to do while caring for a person with dementia, but it's also amazing how rewarding it is to make them feel better."

♦   ♦   ♦

Each time you go to your relative's floor, stop at the nursing station for a brief chat. Greet the nurse on duty by name, and introduce yourself. Ask specific questions, including whether any difficulties have arisen since your last visit and if there is anything you can do to help resolve them.

WHO CAN HELP IF YOU HAVE A PROBLEM?

Roles are very clearly defined in a hospital, but you may not be able to tell a person's job by what he or she is wearing, and you might offend someone by asking him or her the wrong question, or to do something that is not appropriate. For that reason, it is a good idea to acquaint yourself with the responsibilities of each staff member, and to get into the habit of reading everyone's identification tag. That way you will know who is the best person to talk to when you have a problem. The Appendix will provide a description of the roles of the staff members of a hospital.

Keep these questions in mind:

- Who is the best person to ask?
- What is the best way to approach this person?
- How can this person help me get the best care for my relative?
- What does this person need to know about my relative's dementia?

Try to remember that it may take a bit of time to identify the people who can be most helpful to you and to develop a working relationship with them.

◆　◆　◆

Mr. Y had been in the hospital for a few days, when his wife was told that the social worker she had already met with had been transferred to another unit and that a new one had been assigned to the case.

"I was very disappointed that her replacement, who looked very young and inexperienced, and more interested in making a fashion statement than in doing her job, had not made an effort to look at the record. I had already spent a lot of time with the first social worker, and wasn't happy about starting over again with a new person. Besides, I was worried that her apparent lack of concern meant she would not be very helpful. I also thought she was too young to give me the information I needed to take proper care of my husband when he left the hospital. I admit that I got pretty snippy with her."

Rather than continue what she thought was not going to be a productive relationship, Mrs. Y asked to meet with the social work supervisor. She found it more comfortable to communicate with someone in a position of authority, and the two of them quickly worked out the discharge plans.

"Maybe I misjudged the younger social worker, but I knew I wouldn't trust her advice, so I decided to 'go upstairs,' as they say. In some situations, I think you have to go with your gut reaction."

It was very stressful for Mrs. Y to think about taking her husband home from the hospital, and she needed to feel that she was working with someone experienced. "Fortunately, I was able to get my needs met without making a scene."

◆   ◆   ◆

If you are having difficulty deciding when to provide the staff with information and when to let your relative speak for him or herself, it is probably best to give vital information yourself rather than worry about what your relative might have said.

While you will be in constant communication with the staff on your relative's behalf, relationships will develop between members of the staff and the patients for whom they care. You can be supportive of these relationships by staying in the background when it is appropriate.

· 18 ·

How to Make Your Relative More Comfortable in the Hospital Room

Being in a hospital room, with its strange sounds and activities—voices heard over the intercom system, pictures on the wall, the view from the window, the patient in the next bed moaning, screaming, or receiving many telephone calls and visitors—might be upsetting to anyone, but is overwhelming, even terrifying, to a person with Alzheimer's disease.

Dim lighting can cause curtains, furniture, and moving objects to cast frightening shadows. Clutter on the tables or too many chairs and tables will make it hard to get from the bed to the bathroom or even to a nearby chair. Although this confusing environment may cause your relative to become agitated, there are, fortunately, a number of ways to improve the situation.

IN THIS CHAPTER

How Can You Arrange the Hospital Room for a Person with Alzheimer's Disease?

What Are Some Strategies for Managing Common Behavior Problems?

What Can You Do if Your Relative Becomes Agitated?

What If Your Relative Is Verbally or Physically Aggressive?

What Can You Do if Your Relative Has Problems with Other Patients in the Room?

HOW CAN YOU ARRANGE THE HOSPITAL ROOM FOR A PERSON WITH ALZHEIMER'S DISEASE?

It is possible to make changes in your family member's room, within limits. Before doing anything, though, ask the nurse in charge what can be done to comfort your relative. You may also offer suggestions you think might be helpful and see if they are reasonable. The nurse will tell you what can and cannot be changed. Here are some ideas that have worked for other caregivers:

- Look around to see how you can simplify your relative's area of the room. Ask what equipment can be removed, put away in closets, or hidden behind a curtain. Keep items in drawers that your relative does not use all the time.

- Lower the volume on the telephone ringer.

- Ask that the intercom be used as little as possible, or if the volume can be lowered.

- Change the lighting near your relative's bed. Ask if a bright light can be left on.

- Cover or remove pictures.

- Limit the number of visitors.

- If your relative is confused by the view from the window, close the curtains.

- Leave eyeglasses and other essentials within easy reach.

- If your relative has a wheelchair in the room, put it out of the way.

- If possible, push the bed against the wall so your family member can get out on only one side, and you will have more room to move around.

- Close the curtain surrounding the bed to make a more private and secure space for your relative.

- When magazines, leftover juice, and wilting flowers start to accumulate, put the room in order again.

WHAT ARE SOME STRATEGIES FOR MANAGING COMMON BEHAVIOR PROBLEMS?

Your family member is bound to behave in ways that seem problematic in the hospital, although they may have been acceptable at home. If the behavior that is considered "strange" by the staff is not dangerous and will not require more staff time to accommodate, explain that your relative is behaving this way because he or she has dementia, and try to help the staff get into the spirit of going along with it. Some behavior may not be tolerable, however, in which case you may have to intervene.

- If your family member is picking at or pulling out IV lines or other tubes, ask the nurse to place them in a less accessible place (such as high on the dominant arm) or conceal them under the gown.
- If your relative refuses to take a bath, ask the aide to try again at the time he or she is regularly bathed at home, and to respect his or her modesty and privacy as much as possible. If your family member wants to keep his or her clothes on, ask that this be allowed, even though it is not the customary practice.

DEFINITIONS

Agitation: Vocal or motor behavior (screaming, shouting, complaining, moaning, cursing, pacing, fidgeting, wandering, etc.) that is disruptive, unsafe, or interferes with providing care. Agitation in a person with Alzheimer's disease can be a symptom of one or more physical or psychological problems (like pain or depression).

Aggression: Hitting, pushing, or threatening behavior that commonly occurs in a person with Alzheimer's disease when a caregiver attempts to help with daily activities such as dressing.

Disorientation: A cognitive disability in which the senses of time, direction, and thought become confused.

WHAT CAN YOU DO IF YOUR RELATIVE BECOMES AGITATED?

It is possible that your best efforts to keep your family member comfortable and occupied will not prevent him or her from becoming agitated. Sometimes if you just wait, a person with Alzheimer's disease will forget what was so upsetting and calm down. If waiting does not work, consider some of the following suggestions, and try to remain calm yourself.

- Changing the amount of light in the room may be helpful. Experiment with increasing and decreasing the light level to reduce glare and shadows.
- Try to distract your relative by involving him or her in a pleasant activity, such as looking through a magazine, listening to music, folding napkins, or arranging objects on the bed table.
- Seek out special services, such as music, massage, and recreation therapy. Activities and materials for patients with dementia may be available in the hospital.
- If the staff says it is okay, take your relative out of the hospital room. Maybe there is a sunroom or lounge, or you can sit in the lobby for a change of scene.

SUNDOWNING

People with dementia frequently get agitated in the late afternoon and early evening. This is called *sundowning* and results in restless, agitated behavior, and possibly increased wandering or pacing at a time when other people are relaxing and getting ready to eat and go to sleep.

Although no one knows for certain, sundowning may occur because Alzheimer's interferes with the body's clock. It is probably worse when a person is overtired. A short nap early in the afternoon may be helpful. Do not let your relative sleep for too long, though, because a long nap might make it harder to sleep at night.

♦   ♦   ♦

"I don't know who planned this, but did you notice that visiting hours in the hospital and sundowning of AD patients usually happen about the same time?" Frank V said to the social worker, half-jokingly and half-seriously. He had noticed that his wife frequently became agitated in the early evening, just when all the visitors arrived. With four patients in a room, it did not take long for a noisy crowd to gather, and for Mrs. V to start shouting, trying to get out of bed, and rejecting any kind of friendly approach.

The social worker helped Frank make arrangements for his wife to be taken to the garden room before visiting hours began, and for him to visit with her there. This small change worked well for everyone.

♦   ♦   ♦

WHAT IF YOUR RELATIVE IS VERBALLY OR PHYSICALLY AGGRESSIVE?

It is a common myth that all Alzheimer's patients become physically or verbally aggressive. Although this is actually quite unusual, it may occur in the hospital when an individual is more confused and in pain. If your family member is shouting or cursing, you may be very embarrassed, concerned about the reaction of the staff, and worried that something serious is distressing him or her. What can you do?

- You may be able to decrease the aggressive behavior and prevent its recurrence by staying with your relative. Sometimes it is due to fear of being in a strange place, and a familiar face can be calming. (Of course you should stay at a safe distance if your family member is actually trying to hit you.)

- Speak calmly, pat your relative's hand, use reassuring words, offer him or her a treat.

- Do not raise your voice. Your family member will sense your displeasure and may become even more upset.

- Divert your relative by talking about someone who is important to him or her. A picture of a grandchild or something soft to hold might also help.

- Ask the nurse to check if your relative is in pain or has received pain medication.

- If your family member is confined to bed or is unable to walk around, and you are sure he or she is not in pain, try to ignore the behavior. It may help to say that you are going to leave the room until he or she behaves better, and then take a short walk.

- Ask the staff to help you figure out what has caused the outburst. Find out what happened just beforehand. Sometimes a routine event, such as taking temperature or blood pressure, can upset a person with dementia who does not understand what is being done.

- Remind the staff that it is not unusual for patients with AD to react very poorly to being told what to do. They respond better to an invitation than to a command.

- Remember that screaming can be a form of communication for a person who is not able to express feelings adequately with words.

Sometimes people with AD make gestures that seem threatening, like waving their arms, making a fist, or grabbing you. This does not necessarily mean that they are going to become violent. If such behavior has occurred at home, you are probably used to it; but the staff may not be expecting it and fear being hurt. It may help to explain that your relative's "bark is worse than his bite."

If your family member was physically aggressive at home and taking medication for it, tell the doctor. He or she may decide to prescribe the same medication in the hospital. Ask the staff to try to avoid using physical restraints. (For a discussion of restraints, see Chapter 16.)

If your family member is getting very depressed or is often agitated, ask for a psychiatric consultation. Treating depression or anxiety with medication or by changing the environment or daily schedule may ease the distress of the hospitalization.

WHAT ELSE MIGHT BE A PROBLEM?

Some patients with AD begin to think of the hospital as their home. This confusion may result from their poor memory—they have forgotten where they live; or it may be a way of feeling safer and more comfortable—they allow themselves to believe that they are where they want to be.

This belief can be so strong that the person sometimes thinks strangers are entering the room, is unable to understand why they are invading his or her home, and will try to send the other patients' visitors away. If this happens, do not try to convince your relative that he or she is not at home. Instead, explain to the other people in the room that your relative has dementia and really believes that he or she is at home.

Some people with dementia never settle in at all, but repeatedly ask to go home. Although this can be very distressing to you, it may not mean that your relative actually wants to go home, but is expressing discomfort, confusion, or an uneasy feeling that something is wrong.

It may be helpful to respond in a way that lets your family member know that you understand. Try saying something like, "I know you are uncomfortable and want to go home. We'll go as soon as we can." If that doesn't work, try to distract him or her with an activity or by changing the subject.

WHAT CAN YOU DO IF YOUR RELATIVE HAS PROBLEMS WITH OTHER PATIENTS IN THE ROOM?

If your relative is disturbing other patients, let them know that you are aware of the problem and trying to solve it. On the other hand, if you think your relative's roommate is the problem, ask for a different room with a more compatible person. Of course, the other patients may ask for a room change themselves. In the event that your family member cannot tolerate sharing a room with anyone else, consider changing to a private room, even though there will probably be an additional charge.

Remember that your relative is in the hospital for a reason. As important as comfort is, helping him or her cooperate with the medical care is an even greater priority. In the next chapter, we will consider ways you can accomplish this.

· 19 ·

What is Your Role in the Treatment Process?

You can provide a bridge between your anxious relative and the hospital staff whenever he or she has to undergo tests and treatments.. Helping doctors and other staff members communicate with your family member will make it easier for them to treat his or her medical problems. You may also contribute to effective medication management and to reducing the risk of complications of hospitalization to which bedridden patients with dementia are particularly vulnerable.

IN THIS CHAPTER

How Can You Help the Hospital Staff Communicate with Your Family Member?

How Can You Help Your Family Member Cooperate with Medical Care in the Hospital?

What Do You Need to Know about Problems People with Dementia Have with Medication?

What Should You Do if Your Relative Must Stay in Bed?

HOW CAN YOU HELP THE HOSPITAL STAFF COMMUNICATE WITH YOUR FAMILY MEMBER?

Hospital staff members know that it is important to communicate effectively with patients, so it may be necessary to remind them that your relative has Alzheimer's, which makes communicating more difficult. They should also be reminded that the information your relative gives them is often unreliable and, if it has any impact on your relative's health care, should be checked with you.

When staff members are having difficulty communicating with your relative, it may be helpful to mention some of the techniques listed below. They may serve as reminders to you as well, since even if you are used to caring for and communicating with your relative at home, you may feel more uncomfortable and awkward in the hospital, where he or she is more vulnerable, and you are more stressed.

- Approach your relative from the front, get his or her attention, and speak in a soft voice.

- Establish and maintain eye contact.

- Use friendly body language and gentle touch.

- Use simple words and short sentences. Do not overload your family member with information. If his or her attention wanders, gently try to get it back, or wait till later.

- If you cannot understand what your relative is asking for, point to what you think it is, or say the word you believe he or she is trying to find.

- A person with AD may become agitated if he or she has a need—to express pain, for instance—and not be able to tell anyone. Touch the part of the body you think may hurt, and try to tell from his or her facial expression whether that is the problem. If your relative is wiggling, grimacing, or shaking, and you believe he or she may need to go to the bathroom, find someone to take him or her there.

- Avoid questions that your relative cannot answer and may prove embarrassing. Suggest to staff members that rather than ask, "Do you know who I am?" each time they enter the room, say who they are and what they plan to do. For example, "Hi, I'm Milly, and I've come to take your temperature."

- Avoid frustrating your relative by asking him or her to do things that are too difficult. For example, do not give complex instructions that have many steps. Instead, ask him or her to do one thing at a time, show what you want done, and use expressive gestures.

- Be aware of your own body language, tone of voice, and other non-verbal cues. Even a person with advanced dementia can pick up anger, frustration, disgust, impatience, and other negative emotions. If you are losing your patience or cannot keep your emotions in check, take a break. If waiting is not an option, ask someone who is less stressed to talk with your relative for you.

- Above all, do not speak to other people in front of your relative as though he or she were not present. Encourage staff members to include your relative in discussions about his or her medical condition if it is appropriate.

HOW CAN YOU HELP YOUR FAMILY MEMBER COOPERATE WITH MEDICAL CARE IN THE HOSPITAL?

You have probably figured out many ways of helping your family member get through difficult situations. Be sure to tell the staff what has worked before to calm your relative and get his or her cooperation. Ask the staff if you can do anything to help. You may also wish to try the following strategies, which many caregivers have found helpful:

- Be sure you understand the purpose of any planned procedure as well as what it will involve. Will it be painful? Will there be pain or discomfort afterwards? How long will it take? Will it require your relative to lie perfectly still for a long time? Will preparing for the procedure be difficult for a person with AD? For example, will it require swallowing an unpleasant-tasting liquid or having an enema? You may not—and probably will not—wish to tell your family member everything about the procedure, but knowing as much as possible about it yourself will enable you to help both your relative and the staff.

- Wait until shortly before the procedure to tell your relative about it. When information is given too far in advance, it may be forgotten; or the person with AD may ask the same questions over and over or become too anxious to cooperate.

- Explain, if you can, or ask a nurse to explain, one step at a time and in very simple language, what is going to be done or what your relative needs to do.

- Request that procedures be scheduled for a time of day when your family member is most likely to cooperate. Suggest avoiding the late afternoon and evening, when people with AD frequently get agitated and irritable.

- Ask to be with your family member when he or she is being taken (*transported* is the word used in the hospital) from one place to another. He or she will probably be less frightened if you go along.

- Explain to the staff that your relative may be more cooperative if you are allowed to stay during procedures.

- Try to distract your family member while a test or procedure is taking place. This may allow the staff to do its job without interruption.

- If your relative is distressed, ask if it is possible to stop the procedure and allow him or her to calm down before it continues.

- Try to remain as calm as possible. If you feel you cannot, ask another family member or hired helper to take your place, for your relative will only pick up your anxiety and become more anxious.

- If your relative absolutely refuses to do something, wait a few minutes and try again.

◆　　◆　　◆

Ever since the day Mrs. R broke her hip, her son worried that she would not be able to learn to walk again. His concern grew as her stay in the hospital dragged on, and she became more depressed and uncooperative. She began to look like a person with severe AD—much more demented than before she fell. "The antidepressants she was now taking hadn't taken effect, and I was afraid that if she wasn't more willing and able to participate, she would lose her chance to take part in the rehabilitation program at the hospital.

"When the physical therapist from the rehab unit came to evaluate her, I was really upset that my mother would not even try to do anything she was asked to do."

Later in the day, another therapist came to reevaluate Mrs. R when her son was not there. "I think my mother's social self sometimes comes out more when I'm not around. It was lucky that this therapist also had a more engaging manner than the first. Maybe my mother was also more interested in pleasing this therapist because he was a man."

Once Mrs. R was accepted in the rehab program, her son went with her to class. It was obvious that she could not follow the instructions given to the group, or join in the banter the other patients shared. He kept her company while she waited for the therapist to work with her after the class was over. "When it was her turn, I stayed out of her line of vision, so she'd forget I was there. But I did watch so that I would know how to help her later. While it took a lot of my time, I think the investment was worth it."

♦ ♦ ♦

WHAT DO YOU NEED TO KNOW ABOUT PROBLEMS PEOPLE WITH DEMENTIA HAVE WITH MEDICATION?

People with dementia are particularly sensitive to the effects of medication. Special care is required when choosing one, selecting the proper dose and form (liquid, pills, etc.), and deciding how and when it should be given. The inability of people with AD to accurately express their reactions in words makes it all the more important that they be carefully watched so that any side effects, such as changes in behavior or level of confusion, will be noticed at once.

Although your relative's doctor and the hospital staff will be looking out for bad reactions to medication, they may miss signs that you are more likely to notice. They do not know your relative as well as you do, and have many other patients to care for. At such times the one-on-one attention you can give is most valuable. Do not be shy or reluctant to speak up if you notice anything you think might be wrong.

- People with Alzheimer's do feel pain, although they may not say so in conventional ways. If it seems to you that your family member is in pain, ask if and when medication will be given.

- Be sure you know what medications have been prescribed and when your relative is supposed to take them. You should also ask the purpose of each medication when it is given.

- A person with dementia will not be able to tell the doctor about his or her medication history, or bad reactions he or she has had to medications in the past, so you will have to. If you have filled out the *Profile of the Person with Memory Impairment* (see Chapter 7), you may want to look it over to remind yourself.

- People with dementia may have paradoxical reactions to medications, which means that the medicine has an effect that is opposite from what is generally expected. For example, a medicine meant to calm may cause agitation, or a medicine meant to help your relative sleep may cause insomnia instead. If you find him or her very confused and upset, ask the doctor to reevaluate the prescribed medications.

- When a new medicine is prescribed, inquire about its side effects. Many drugs can increase confusion or interfere with balance, which might result in a fall.

- Some people hate to take pills. If the medication cannot be given in any other form, tell the staff how you get your relative to take pills at home. Maybe you have found that crushing them in apple sauce or dissolving them in juice works best.

- Sometimes people with AD will insist on holding and playing with their pills until some or all fall on the floor. Or they might hold the pill in their mouth and then spit it out when no one is looking. Ask whoever is giving the pills to hand them over one at a time and make sure each is swallowed.

- Do not give your relative medicine from home. While in the hospital, patients should only take medicines prescribed by hospital doctors and only on the hospital's schedule.

WHAT SHOULD YOU DO IF YOUR RELATIVE
MUST STAY IN BED?

People with Alzheimer's are very vulnerable to physical decline caused by immobility. When a person is kept in bed and does not move around, muscles quickly begin to tighten. Range-of-motion exercises, which gently move each joint, can prevent this loss of flexibility and the development of a more serious condition of the joints called *contracture*, which can be painful and make caregiving more difficult. One of your daily tasks will be to make sure that your relative is up and about as much as his or her condition allows, and that he or she receives the appropriate exercises. If your family member is not getting physical therapy, ask the doctor if he will recommend it.

The chance that an Alzheimer's patient will fall is greater if muscle tone has been lost as a result of spending a great deal of time in bed. The risk is increased by the side effects of certain medications, which interfere with balance, and from the neurological symptoms of AD. If your family member is distracted and in an unfamiliar environment, he or she may easily trip. For all these reasons, a person with AD needs to be closely watched in the hospital.

Pressure or bed sores are another problem that can develop from staying in bed and not being able to move. They are more likely to develop if a person is poorly nourished. These very painful wounds result from pressure on sensitive skin; they can be prevented by turning or moving the person frequently, and assuring an adequate diet. Materials such as lambs wool and "egg crate" foam pads to prevent rubbing against the sheets or chair can also reduce the chance that these sores will develop.

People who need to stay in bed, especially if they are elderly, are often put in diapers or have a catheter inserted for urination. If possible, try to avoid the use of a catheter, which sometimes leads to urinary tract infections and might be pulled out by a confused patient. If your relative was able to use the toilet before coming to the hospital, ask the staff to let him or her do so again as soon as possible. You do not want the habit to be lost.

The more you can do to help your family member cooperate with care in the hospital, the better the chances that you will be able to bring him or her home relatively soon. As your relative gets closer to the end of the hospitalization, your next task will be to address his or her future care needs.

·20·

Preparing for Discharge from the Hospital

With length of hospital stays decreased and many tests performed on an outpatient basis, patients are being discharged as soon as they are medically stable, although they may still need a great deal of care. Since people with Alzheimer's disease generally take longer to get better after an illness than other elderly people, they may not function as well after a hospital stay as they did before. With good care and the passage of time, however, many of them will recover.

You, as caregiver, will play an important role in planning for the care of your relative after he or she leaves the hospital. The more you know about what a *discharge plan* may and should include, the better you will be able to prepare for the next step in caring for your family member with Alzheimer's.

IN THIS CHAPTER

What Is a Discharge Plan and How Is It Developed?

What Does a Discharge Plan Include?

Where Will Your Relative Go After the Hospital Stay?

WHAT IS A DISCHARGE PLAN AND HOW IS IT DEVELOPED?

A discharge plan contains recommendations that will ensure the ongoing care of a patient upon leaving the hospital. It may call for services to be provided in your or your relative's home, or somewhere more appropriate to his or her needs at the time of discharge.

Although you will probably not be aware of it, discharge planning begins the moment a patient enters the hospital (or even before, if it's a planned hospitalization). The medical team continually watches for changes in your relative's medical condition and ability to function so that an appropriate discharge plan will be prepared when he or she is ready to leave the hospital.

The plan will be based on the patient's medical needs, as well as benefits covered by insurance, and how much can be paid for privately. It will take into consideration information from you about how much help the family will be able to provide, and the physical conditions where your relative will be living—for example, whether or not there are stairs. You may have had help in caring for your relative at home before the hospitalization, but upon returning, he or she will probably, at least temporarily, need more.

The discharge plan is created under the supervision of the doctor responsible for your relative's hospital care. Its primary consideration is the patient's safety. If you disagree with the discharge date or believe your relative needs care that can be provided only in the hospital, discuss it with the doctor. It may be useful to have the patient's primary care physician, even if he has not been involved in the hospitalization, speak to him as well. If these steps are unsuccessful, you can, as a last resort, appeal the discharge plan.

Before your relative leaves the hospital, the discharge plan will be reviewed with you, so you should certainly speak up if anything else about it does not seem workable. When your relative is ready to leave the hospital, you will be given a written copy of the plan and prescriptions for new medications.

WHAT DOES A DISCHARGE PLAN INCLUDE?

The discharge plan will include a recommendation about where your relative will receive after care, as well as the kinds of services he or she will get and from whom. The services of a home health aide, nurse, physical therapist, occupational therapist, speech therapist, and social worker may all be part of the discharge plan, and can be provided either at home or in another health care facility. Equipment and supplies needed during recovery will be ordered for your relative if he or she is going home.

◆　　◆　　◆

"I was really offended when the social worker at the hospital suggested that my wife should go to a nursing home and not back home with me when her treatment was finished," said Mr. D. "I didn't think she was that bad, and I had promised her when she was first diagnosed with Alzheimer's disease that I would always take care of her."

The social worker in the hospital pointed out that neither of them was as healthy as they were when that promise had been made, and that the stress of caring for Mrs. D might be too much for her husband now. "I have to admit that sometimes when I am very tired and not sure what to do for my wife, I wonder how much longer I can go on this way. But I don't let myself think about this for long. And I never say it to my children.

"Well, I took my wife back home again, but I didn't forget everything the social worker had said." Mrs. D has been enrolled in an adult day care program for people with dementia, and Mr. D asks his grown children to help out on the weekend. "I realize that someday it may be best for all of us if my wife were in a nursing home. I'm looking around now just in case it has to happen, and believe me, I'll find the best one."

◆　　◆　　◆

WHAT SERVICES WILL BE COVERED BY INSURANCE?

Health insurers impose restrictions on what can be offered to the people they insure. The fact that your family member has AD does not mean that extra days in the hospital or increased home care services will be covered. The number of hours of home care and the types and amount of equipment and supplies that are offered are also restricted by the insurance plan.

Discharge planners will review your relative's insurance benefits and discuss how many of the services he or she needs are covered. They will know how much physical or occupational therapy the insurance company will pay for. Insurance companies may question a dementia patient's ability to participate fully in rehabilitation or to benefit from it.

If you feel that a service such as physical therapy has been unfairly rejected because he or she has AD, this is the time to advocate for your family member. It may help your case to assure the planner, who is in contact with the insurance company, that you will watch the therapist work with your relative, and will help him or her maintain between sessions the skills that have been taught.

WHERE WILL YOUR RELATIVE GO
AFTER THE HOSPITAL STAY?

Hospital discharge planners may believe that a nursing home is the appropriate place for people with dementia, but this is not necessarily true. In many cases a person can return home after a hospitalization if the family is willing and able to provide care. Even if you have no intention of placing your family member in a nursing home, try not to be upset by the suggestion. It does not mean you are doing a bad job of caregiving. The staff just wants to make sure that you are aware of your options. You may feel able and willing to continue caring for your family member at home. Ultimately, the decision is up to you. Remember that any plan can be changed, and that your relative can leave one facility and receive care in another setting.

If you choose to have your relative move in with you, there will be new and different demands on your time, and you may have to rearrange your home to make room for your family member. But if you have been traveling long distances to visit and worrying in between, this arrangement may actually make things easier for you.

It is possible that the discharge planner will recommend that your relative be transferred to another facility, either for a short stay or on a permanent basis. In the chapters that follow, we will discuss each of these alternatives in greater detail. Whether your relative goes home or to another facility, the process of recovery should be supported by the services in the discharge plan.

After a hospitalization, things may return to normal—or as close to normal as living with AD can ever be—or they may change in small and large ways. You may have to help your family member make the transition to a different living arrangement while adjusting to the changes in circumstances yourself.

PART FOUR

♦ ♦ ♦

After the Hospital

· 21 ·

When Your Relative Is Discharged Home

You probably have been looking forward to the time when your family member leaves the hospital and both of you can get back to your usual routine. After your relative's medical condition has been treated and he or she is feeling better, things may get back to normal very quickly, but in the event that he or she has become more frail or confused as a result of the hospitalization, or needs rehabilitation after discharge, you may be faced with new problems to solve.

IN THIS CHAPTER

How Can You Prepare the Home for Your Relative's Return?

What Kinds of Services Will Your Family Member Get at Home?

What If Your Relative Needs Complicated Medical Equipment or Treatment after Discharge?

What If Additional Home Care Is Needed?

What If It Becomes Too Difficult to Care for Your Relative at Home?

HOW CAN YOU PREPARE THE HOME FOR YOUR RELATIVE'S RETURN?

Changes may have to be made at home so that it will be easier for your family member to get around and for you to give the necessary care. Doing this beforehand will allow you to be and less frazzled at the time of discharge and more available to help him or her make the transition. Here are some suggestions:

- Stock up on basic home and medical supplies.
- Fill new prescriptions.
- Have new equipment delivered and installed.

In addition, certain changes can make the home more convenient and safe.

- If the rooms are cluttered, rearrange the furniture and remove unnecessary objects so that it is easy for your relative to move around safely.
- If your relative has trouble climbing stairs or getting to the bathroom, move him or her to a room that is on the same floor as and closer to the bathroom.
- Be sure that he or she can get from room to room, especially into the bathroom; you may have to remove doors to permit a wheelchair or walker to get through.
- Check out the safety of the home again, with a view toward your relative's new needs and the convenience of caregiving.

♦ ♦ ♦

"When I took my mother home after six weeks in the hospital she was an entirely different person than before she broke her hip," Mary P said. Her mother seemed depressed and much more confused.

"While she was in the hospital, she asked, literally hundreds of times, 'When am I going home.' But when she finally got here, she expressed no joy. In fact, she didn't even recognize the place. Even though I had been

warned that this might happen, I guess I secretly hoped it wouldn't be true."
Mary felt disappointed and pessimistic about the future.

She had made what she thought was every preparation possible for her
mother's return. "The guard rails were finally on the bed (after two
appointments for delivery had been broken), and the furniture had been
slightly rearranged to make a clear passage to the bathroom. Only when we
got home did I realize that the wheelchair would not fit through the bath-
room door." Mary ended up hiring a carpenter to remove the bathroom
door and replace it with double doors with hinges outside the frame so the
wheelchair would pass through.

She also had hired an aide for the night shift to ensure her mother's
safety. "You won't believe this, but while the aide was in the kitchen
making her tea, my mother, who could barely move, slipped out through
the tiny space between the end of the guard rail and the bookcase that
had been placed next to her bed and went to the bathroom. I would have
sworn that a mouse couldn't have gotten through that space. It was a mir-
acle that she managed to do this without hurting herself again. After that
I just left the rail down. It seemed better than having her climb over or
squeeze around it."

Mary knows it is impossible to completely protect a person who is no
longer able to understand when she is putting herself in danger, but she
believes that all her preparations and precautions gave her mother the best
chance to recover. Within a few months. Mrs. P did get much better. She
was never the same as before she had fallen, but she got around fairly well
and felt comfortable at home again.

♦   ♦   ♦

It is natural to expect your family member to be pleased at being back
home. Try not to be disappointed and angry if this doesn't happen. When
the dementia is severe, and the hospitalization has been long, your relative
may no longer remember his or her home, even if it has not been changed
at all. A person with dementia will need time and help to readjust because
home will seem like a new environment.

WHAT KINDS OF SERVICES WILL
YOUR RELATIVE GET AT HOME?

If your family member goes home, the discharge plan can include:

- Nursing supervision.
- Home health aide(s).
- Therapists (physical, occupational, speech).
- A social worker.
- Equipment.

Most insurance plans, including Medicare and Medicaid (or state-funded insurance plans), will pay for a few hours a day of care at home by a home health aide for as long as there is a medical need. The discharge planner will generally provide the family with a list of licensed agencies that offer home care services. The agency you choose will make the final decision about the services the patient is qualified to receive, and will accept a plan only if it believes it is safe and will work.

HOME CARE AGENCIES

Agencies differ in the range of services they offer and the fees they charge. Some require that you pay them; and they, in turn, will pay the home care personnel. They also usually handle the paperwork for their employees, including taxes and insurance. A number of them, CHHAs (Certified Home Health Agencies), provide services that can be reimbursed by Medicare, Medicaid, and other third-party insurance; while others, licensed by individual states, can offer home care services to people who qualify for Medicaid. Each state has its own Medicaid requirements and provides different amounts of care to eligible clients.

In addition, there are private home health agencies that are not eligible for insurance reimbursement because they are not regulated or licensed. Some of these screen their employees, though you may want to check their references yourself. If you use one of these agencies, it will pay the workers, and you will pay the agency.

Registries serve as employment agencies for home care personnel. They are not required to screen or background check the personnel, although some do. You pay a fee to the agency, employ the person directly, and are responsible for payroll taxes and Social Security.

The hospital can recommend agencies that offer the services you need. You might also find people to provide these services by asking other caregivers how they got help. Someone else who has been in your position may know exactly what you need.

NURSING SUPERVISION. Home care services provided by a Certified Home Health Agency are supervised by a visiting nurse, who periodically checks on the patient. The nurse, who is employed by the agency, not the hospital, can help you with medical equipment, make sure you are using it correctly, and report changes in your relative's condition to the primary care physician. He or she also determines the number of hours of home care the agency provides, and ultimately decides when the home care service will be terminated.

HOME HEALTH AIDES can help patients with bathing, dressing, eating, walking around the house, and going to the bathroom. Although they are not responsible for cooking and cleaning, they can prepare a meal or change bed linens when no one from the family is available. They cannot, however, administer medications or provide any medical care or assistance with surgical dressings.

REHABILITATION THERAPY. If the discharge plan includes physical and/or occupational therapy, a therapist will visit the home to work with your relative. It will be a good idea for you to observe and possibly participate in therapy sessions so you can practice the exercises and activities when the therapist is not there, either between sessions or after therapeutic services end. As with a home health aide, ask for someone who has experience with AD. Insurance provides rehabilitation only as long as the patient continues to make progress. You may decide to pay for additional rehabilitation to maintain your relative's ability to function. These extra services may improve your relative's quality of life and make your caregiving task easier.

WHO PROVIDES REHABILITATION?

If your relative is scheduled to receive physical, occupational, or speech therapy at home, what can you expect these therapists to do?

Physical therapists help a person regain strength and movement after an illness or injury. They teach people to use devices such as crutches, walkers, or grab bars, and how to do special exercises.

Occupational therapists help people re-learn the skills of everyday life, such as eating and dressing, when doing these tasks have been affected by illness or injury.

Speech therapists help people with their language and communication problems, as well as swallowing difficulties.

EQUIPMENT. Every effort will be made to ensure that the home environment is safe. The discharge planner will order the necessary equipment to be delivered to your relative's home. This might include a wheelchair, walker, raised toilet seat, shower bench, and grab bars for the shower or tub, as well as a special bed, rubber sheets, portable commode, and various other devices. Some of these will be authorized and paid for by the insurance company because they are needed for the home care of your relative on discharge from the hospital. You may, however, feel it is necessary to purchase additional items that are not covered by your relative's insurance, such as an electrically powered chair to help him or her get up from a seated position.

If at all possible, have the new equipment delivered and installed before your relative gets home. This will ease the transition from hospital to home and give you one less thing to worry about. Some of this equipment may have to be returned when no longer considered necessary, although in general, arrangements can be made for you to buy these items if you think they are still needed.

WHAT IF YOUR RELATIVE NEEDS COMPLICATED MEDICAL EQUIPMENT OR TREATMENT AFTER DISCHARGE?

Patients are frequently discharged from the hospital while they are still using complicated devices such as catheters, feeding tubes, and respirators, or need wound care. You or another family member may have to learn to use new and unfamiliar medical equipment at home. It is essential that you be trained to do this while your relative is still in the hospital. Sometimes equipment ordered for home use differs slightly from the kind used in the hospital. Ask if it is possible to be trained on exactly the same model of the equipment you will be using at home. It is important that you feel confident in your ability to use medical equipment safely on your own. Be sure to get the telephone number of the company that distributes the device, and find out the kind of support services it offers. You will also need to learn to recognize the signs of infections and other complications of your relative's medical condition, and when you should seek professional help to treat them.

Most agencies do not train or permit home health aides to use medical equipment. Since the nurse cannot be there all the time, you may be expected to monitor treatments and machines on which your relative's life depends. This may seem like a huge and terrifying responsibility, especially when your family member first comes home. You may not feel confident that you will be able to handle all that is expected. When this happens, and you feel that you need more training, you can ask the company that sent the equipment to send someone to your home to show you how to use it until you feel comfortable. You can also request additional support from the nurse during his or her regular visits. If you need more help from the nurse than the insurance covers, you may need to pay for it privately.

WHAT IF ADDITIONAL HOME CARE IS NEEDED?

Home care covered by insurance is linked to the need for skilled nursing care. When the nurse is no longer required, other services are also stopped. This does not necessarily mean that the patient is not in need of further care. An issue of major concern to family caregivers of someone with AD is long-term custodial care after the acute condition has been resolved, since it is neither provided by Medicare nor most insurance companies unless your relative has purchased long-term care insurance.

DEFINITIONS

Activities of daily living (ADLs): Include eating, bathing, dressing, toileting, bowel and bladder control, and getting in and out of a chair.

Custodial care (sometimes called *personal care*): The provider, who does not need to have medical skills, helps a person perform the activities of daily living.

Skilled nursing care: Care is considered skilled when a trained professional, such as a registered nurse or professional therapist, must do it.

If you think your relative needs more professional home care and supervision than is provided by insurance, these are some options to consider. You can pay for it yourself, although you may need to use a different agency than the one included in the discharge plan. Home health aides can come from an agency or be hired privately. When you hire someone privately, you will be responsible for finding a replacement if you are dissatisfied or the aide is unable to be there. An agency will probably try to find someone who works well with you and your relative, send that person regularly, and provide a substitute when the regular person is not available. Ask for aides who are skilled at working with people with Alzheimer's. There are now agencies that offer special training in Alzheimer's care.

Alternatively, you and your family may decide to provide extra care for your relative with AD yourselves. In that case, try to work out a schedule that does not put too much of a burden on any single individual. If your relative is physically well enough, a day care center may offer supervision and social contact, while giving the family a needed respite. Other family caregivers at the hospital or the hospital social worker may be able to tell you how to find the resources you need.

◆   ◆   ◆

Before Mr. K went into the hospital, his wife had gotten him on a schedule for going to the bathroom, taking him every two hours. "If he needed to go at another time, I could usually tell by the way he would wiggle around and get kind of nervous. When he was in the hospital, though, they put him in what they call 'diapers,' (a word that always upset me, so I asked them not to say 'diapers' in front of him). I had no idea that he would not remember how to use the bathroom when he got home. I couldn't bear it. Maybe I was still exhausted from the whole hospitalization experience, or maybe the fact that my daughter, who was always so supportive, had to move far away because her husband got a new job, but I just could not think about changing Joe as if he were a baby. Maybe it just hurt me too much to see him that way."

She spoke to her daughter, and they decided it would be best for Mr. K to be placed in a nursing home at this point. Then she could visit him as well as her daughter, whom she missed a lot, without having to worry about who would take care of him. "It wasn't an easy decision, but I think it was the best one for us."

◆   ◆   ◆

WHAT IF IT BECOMES TOO DIFFICULT TO CARE FOR YOUR RELATIVE AT HOME?

The experience of caring for your relative at home may be very different from the way it was before he or she went into the hospital. The dementia may have become more severe, and your relative may require more care. It may be too frightening or burdensome for you to manage the responsibility of what may be life-sustaining equipment. There may be other caregiving tasks that you find you cannot tolerate. Despite your efforts to adjust to the new demands, you may realize that you can no longer care for him or her at home. In this case, you may wish to consider placing your relative in a subacute-care facility or nursing home on a temporary or permanent basis. (Some alternatives are discussed in the next chapter).

· 22 ·

If Your Relative Cannot Go Directly Home

A hospital stay is often a turning point in the life of a person with Alzheimer's. It almost always leads to changes in the person and the way caregivers view his or her needs as well as their own. Even if your relative's condition has not worsened in the hospital, seeing the situation through the perspective of the staff may make it clear to you that he or she can no longer live at home.

The hospital discharge plan will include a recommendation for a facility that will meet your relative's care needs. Among the possibilities are *subacute-care facilities*, which provide short-term medical care, *nursing homes*, for people who require medical care on a more permanent basis, and *residential care facilities*, for those needing supervision or help with the activities of daily living. The discharge planner will work with you to find a suitable place.

IN THIS CHAPTER

Where Can a Person Get Short-Term Care after a Hospital Stay?

What If Nursing Home Placement Is Recommended?

What Other Living Arrangements Are Available for a Person with Alzheimer's Disease?

> What Should You Look for in a Facility?
> How Can You and Your Relative Adjust to the Change in Living Arrangements?

WHERE CAN A PERSON GET SHORT-TERM CARE AFTER A HOSPITAL STAY?

After a hospitalization, many people need ongoing care, which, for a variety of reasons, cannot be provided at home. Those who can benefit from many hours a day of intensive physical rehabilitation, for instance, will be referred to a facility designed exclusively for this purpose. People with AD, however, may not be able to follow instructions, participate in group activities, or tolerate such a rigorous program. In that case, a subacute-care facility may be more appropriate for their needs, enabling them to receive rehabilitation at a slower pace. These facilities also provide skilled short-term nursing care (such as changing a dressing on a wound) for those who are medically stable.

Caregivers may be reluctant to send a person with dementia to a sub-acute-care facility, however, since it is often located in a nursing home; and the idea of going there, even for a short time, may be frightening to caregiver and patient alike. Another worry is that their family member will not be able to adjust to another new setting, or that he or she will never come home again, so they may take him or her directly home despite the difficulty of providing the necessary care. Before you decide, visit the facility recommended by the hospital, and talk to the staff as well as to caregivers of other facility residents.

◆　　◆　　◆

Mr. G was in the mild stage of AD and living alone. His brother Martin would look in on him every day to see how he was doing and cook him a hot meal. "We were managing pretty well until he had a small stroke and went to the hospital. The combination of stroke and AD really hit him hard," Martin said.

When it was time to leave the hospital, the social worker recommended that Mr. G go to a subacute-care facility. "Well, I had never heard of that, and neither had my brother. She explained that it was a place where he would be cared for while getting the physical therapy he needed. It was frightening to me because it was actually in the wing of a nursing home, but since it wasn't too far from where we lived, I went to look at the place. It was clean, and I saw that people like him were doing special exercises. I knew that he couldn't go back home the way he was, and so he and I agreed that going to this place would be the best plan."

◆   ◆   ◆

WHAT IF NURSING HOME PLACEMENT IS RECOMMENDED?

A nursing home (or skilled nursing facility) is a place that gives nursing care, help with healing after an injury or hospital stay, or custodial care. It is not uncommon for the health care team to suggest that a person with dementia go to a nursing home at the end of a hospital stay, even though the person may have been living at home before entering the hospital. The team may feel that he or she needs more care as a result of the recent illness than can be provided at home.

Some caregivers are relieved that someone else has suggested nursing home placement. They may feel guilty even thinking about it, and welcome help in taking this step. A hospitalization can provide you with an opportunity to look more objectively at your relative's situation and your ability to continue to provide care.

Even caregivers who have a firm commitment to home care may find at some point that they are not able or no longer choose to keep their relative at home. They may be exhausted or ill or have other obligations in their lives that require attention. A nursing home may be an appropriate choice. It may, in fact, be the best choice if your relative with Alzheimer's disease needs round-the-clock care or ongoing medical treatment.

Most nursing homes have services and staff to address issues such as medical care, nutrition, recreation, and spirituality. Many have special care units designed to meet the unique needs of people with dementia. If you are considering nursing home placement, it will be necessary to visit several homes to get a sense of how they differ and which will best meet your relative's needs.

WHAT OTHER LIVING ARRANGEMENTS ARE AVAILABLE FOR A PERSON WITH ALZHEIMER'S DISEASE?

If the discharge plan does not indicate the need for a skilled nursing facility, or the family and patient oppose nursing home placement, a variety of supportive housing alternatives, providing different levels of care, are available. Some of these facilities are covered by insurance, although most are not.

DEFINITIONS

Congregate housing: Offers a minimum service package that includes some meals served in a common dining room, and may offer on-site medical/nursing services, personal care, or housekeeping.

Group home and board-and-care residences: Provide residential-type accommodations, personal services, and opportunities for socializing for people who are not related to the owner and do not have an illness, which requires regular medical care or twenty-four-hour nursing services.

Assisted or sheltered housing: Generally offers a more extensive package of services, with emphasis on meals, personal care, and social activities. The staff helps residents with dressing, bathing, feeding, and housekeeping. However, a less-skilled level of care is provided than in a nursing home.

Retirement housing: Generally provides each resident with an apartment or room that includes cooking facilities. Since the staff may have little or no knowledge about dementia, and is usually not available around the clock, this setting may be appropriate for people in the early stage of Alzheimer's who can still care for themselves and live alone safely, but have difficulty managing an entire house.

Continuum of care retirement communities (CCRC): Provide all of the options described above. In these facilities, a person may receive all levels of care on one campus, but may have to be moved to a different building when additional services are needed.

In the private sector, there are senior residences and assisted (or enriched) living facilities as well as board-and-care facilities, which offer services for elders with dementia. Most of these places, however, are not monitored by regulatory agencies, and are geared to relatively high-functioning and independent older people who may have some minor care needs. Their prices differ, but they generally attract people with financial means.

There are also group homes, adult homes, and other types of congregate housing that have financial eligibility criteria and provide a wide range of services, usually including security, on-site meals served in a common dining room, housekeeping, and social activities. Some also offer on-site nursing services.

There is probably a facility in your area that meets your relative's needs. Before you decide, though, visit the one recommended by the hospital. Talk to the staff as well as to residents and their caregivers. Of course, your relative's particular needs will determine the kind of facility you choose.

WHAT SHOULD YOU LOOK FOR IN A FACILITY?

There is much you can discover about a particular facility before visiting it. A hospital social worker can guide you and recommend many books that will tell you what to look for. If you are not satisfied with what you have learned, keep on searching until you find the place that best fits your relative's needs as well as yours. Here are some questions to ask:

- What kind of resident are they designed to serve?
- What provisions or services do they offer, specifically for people with Alzheimer's disease?
- Can they provide care over the entire course of the disease? If not, at what point in the course of AD would a resident have to leave?
- What services are included in the fee? What do you have to pay extra for?
- Can additional services be brought in, or does the resident have to move out if more care is needed?
- What happens when the person can no longer pay?

- Is there any financial penalty for leaving?
- Is the facility covered by any regulations, and if so, has it been cited for violations?
- Is it conveniently located so that family and friends can visit?
- What is the staff-to-resident ratio?
- What medical coverage is available at the residence? Is a nurse always on the site? Is there a specific doctor who visits the facility? Can your relative continue to use his or her own doctor? Where do they send patients if hospitalization is needed?
- What are the arrangements for giving medication?
- What training does the staff receive?
- Can personal possessions be brought to the facility?
- Does this facility meet any religious requirements that your relative may have?

While you can learn a great deal by asking questions on the telephone and reading brochures, there are some things you can find out only by visiting:

- How clean is it?
- Are most of the residents engaged in activities?
- Do staff and residents seem to interact well with each other?
- Do you see residents receiving the kind of rehabilitation the hospital is recommending for your relative?

HOW CAN YOU AND YOUR RELATIVE ADJUST TO THE CHANGE IN LIVING ARRANGEMENTS?

You may have to help your family member make the transition to a different living arrangement while adjusting to the changes in your own circumstances. At first, you and other family members may be the only familiar people in your relative's life. It will help if you bring a few favorite items to put in his or her room.

You can help the staff of the facility understand your family member's needs and strengths by giving an up-to-date copy of the *Profile of a Person with Memory Impairment* to the person most responsible for the care of your relative.

Nursing homes and assisted living facilities generally have support groups to help caregivers adjust to their family member's absence from home. They will also help you develop working relationships with the staff of the facility.

In the course of being a caregiver for a relative with Alzheimer's disease, you have had to make many decisions and adjust to many changes. While you may have fewer hands-on tasks to perform now that your relative is no longer living at home, you will still be a very important part of his or her life.

· 23 ·

The Death of a Person with Alzheimer's Disease

There is a growing appreciation in the medical community that the final phase of life can be very meaningful for all concerned. When someone has been suffering from Alzheimer's disease over many years, the process of letting go and saying good-bye may have been taking place in steps as the disease has progressed.

Caregivers will sometimes be faced with important decisions on their relative's behalf as death draws near, such as whether to allow doctors to try to prolong his or her life and when to withhold or withdraw treatment.

IN THIS CHAPTER

What Will You Do When Your Relative's Death Is Near?

How Can You Follow Your Relative's Advance Directives?

What Is Palliative Care?

What Is Hospice Care?

Should Your Relative Receive Palliative Care?

What Should You Do When Your Relative Dies?

Should an Autopsy of Your Relative's Brain Be Performed?

And now, You. . .

WHAT WILL YOU DO WHEN YOUR
RELATIVE'S DEATH IS NEAR?

During the long course of AD, patients may develop other illnesses that will eventually cause their death. This requires caregivers and physicians to consider both the person's stage of dementia and medical condition when making decisions about care for him or her in the final phase of life.

Some people with AD may live until the last stage of the disease and then die from a total collapse of mind and body. When people die in the severe stage of dementia without any other medical illness, it generally appears as a slow shutting down of all systems. Sometimes pneumonia or another infection is the immediate cause of death at this late stage.

People have very intense and conflicting feelings about what should be done for a dying person. For some, it is important that death be as natural as possible. Others prefer to use the many medical methods that are now available to extend the lives of the gravely ill. Mechanical devices such as feeding tubes and respirators may be routinely used in some settings. In others, they may be viewed as inappropriate for elderly people, particularly those with dementia. These methods are sometimes referred to by those who oppose them as tools to extend the dying process.

HOW CAN YOU FOLLOW YOUR
RELATIVE'S ADVANCE DIRECTIVES?

If your relative is in a nursing home or hospital, find out if its policies will allow it to carry out your relative's wishes as expressed in the advance directives. It may be associated with a religious organization that prevents it from honoring those wishes. If that is the case, you may decide to make arrangements to transfer your relative to another institution.

If you and your relative have agreed in advance that all end-of-life care will be provided at home, consult with his or her doctor about what medical conditions will be treated aggressively, and when only palliative care will be given. Ask your relative's doctor whether he or she will help you carry out your relative's wishes for care through the dying process. You may wish to consider enrolling your relative in a hospice program (which is described below). You do not need a referral from a physician to obtain hospice services, but can contact your local hospice program directly. It will send a staff member to determine your relative's suitability for this service. Such programs can be found through your local hospital, the Yellow Pages of your telephone book, or the National Hospice Association, which is included in the Appendix. Hospice services are covered by Medicare and Medicaid.

WHAT IS PALLIATIVE CARE?

Palliative care is a branch of medicine that not only treats the medical needs of those living with terminal illness, but also includes their family and friends in their care. Its aim is not to cure, but to give the patient the best possible quality of life.

It can be started at any point toward the end of life, at home or in a hospital, and signals a shift in goals from active treatment to supportive care, including services designed to relieve pain, reduce stress, and provide emotional support, information, and referrals for both the patient and family members.

If the hospital where your relative is being treated has a palliative care program, a physician, nurse, or social worker can refer you and your relative for its services. Your relative's insurance may or may not cover the cost of palliative care, so this is something to investigate before making a decision.

WHAT IS HOSPICE CARE?

Hospice care is a form of palliative care specifically designed for the very last months of life. Patients can be transferred to hospice care when their physicians believe they have six or fewer months to live.

In a hospice program, doctors, nurses, social workers, home health aides, clergy, and volunteers guide and support the patient and family in coping with medical, psychological, and spiritual needs. They focus on keeping the patient comfortable by managing pain and symptoms. These services are generally provided in the home, but may also be offered in a special area of a hospital or in a nursing home. After the patient dies, bereavement and other services are available to the family.

There is, unfortunately, a lot of misunderstanding about when and whether hospice care is appropriate. Doctors may be reluctant to give up trying to cure their patients even when there is almost no chance of success; families may also want the doctors to keep trying. In most cases when death is inevitable, a hospice offers the kinds of medical care and supportive services that the dying and their family members need.

Guidelines have been developed to help physicians and family members decide whether referral to this valuable service is appropriate. A maximum six-month life expectancy is the formal requirement, largely because of Medicare regulations. People with Alzheimer's are eligible when they have an acute illness and are in the final stage of AD.

SHOULD YOUR RELATIVE RECEIVE PALLIATIVE CARE?

When and if you come to understand and accept that curative treatment is no longer available or desirable, this does not mean that nothing can be done for your relative. At this time patients and their families still need, and should expect, respectful, kind, and supportive services.

Whether the primary medical problem is related to Alzheimer's or another chronic illness, palliative or hospice care can provide comfort to the dying person and his or her family when a decision has been made to stop aggressive treatment. This makes it possible for the family of a dying person to feel that instead of withholding treatment, they are giving their family member with Alzheimer's the best possible care until the last moment of life.

WHAT SHOULD YOU DO WHEN YOUR RELATIVE DIES?

If your relative dies in the hospital or under hospice care at home, arrangements will be made for the disposition of the body. When he or she dies at home and is not receiving hospice care, each locality has its own procedure. It generally includes calling 911. The police may come to the house and then contact the medical examiner, who will determine whether to send an investigator or make arrangements with your relative's doctor to sign a death certificate. The next step is for the funeral home to be contacted. A local funeral home or the medical examiner can provide specific guidelines for your area.

SHOULD AN AUTOPSY OF YOUR RELATIVE'S BRAIN BE PERFORMED?

At the time of your relative's death, it may be very hard to think about whether or not to have an autopsy performed. It is easier to think about an autopsy in advance and discuss it with family members and your relative when he or she is still able to participate in making the decision. Some people, upon learning that they have Alzheimer's disease, request that an autopsy be performed when they die. If that is the case with your relative, it should be included in his or her advance directives, and you should be guided by these wishes.

Some families request an autopsy to confirm the cause of death. Another reason is a desire to contribute to knowledge about Alzheimer's disease. An autopsy of the brain does not disfigure the body; and a funeral, even with an open casket, can be held without delay.

If you or your family member wants an autopsy performed, inform your relative's doctor, other family members, and the funeral home of the plan. In many locales the medical examiner can arrange for one, often free of charge. Alternatively, your relative's doctor may have the hospital with which he is affiliated perform the autopsy. As with all these arrangements, it is a good idea to find out in advance what the policy is where your relative lives. If he or she has been enrolled in a research program that makes autopsy arrangements, contact the coordinator. If you are being urged by hospital personnel to allow an autopsy, but you or your family are opposed, you have the right, in most cases, to decline.

◆　　◆　　◆

After putting it off for months, Diane and her husband Mark had finally gotten away for a weekend, leaving Mark's mother Jenny, who had moderately severe AD, at home with her favorite aide Marie. Jenny waved them off when they left, seeming in better spirits and health than she had been of late.

"When I answered the phone early Sunday morning and heard Marie's familiar voice, I was completely unprepared for her words, 'Jenny's dead.' I really had no idea what to do or say."

Diane and Mark immediately drove to Jenny's house. "I don't know what I thought would happen next, but I was completely taken aback to find two policemen sitting in the living room along with Jenny's niece Ruth and my friend Isabel, who had often visited with Jenny. It never occurred to me that Jenny's body would still be in her bed, where she had died. The policemen, who were very kind, told us that certain forms needed to be completed before the body could be released to the funeral parlor."

Someone had already contacted Jenny's doctor, who had treated her heart problems for years, and asked him to sign the death certificate. Diane and Mark were overwhelmed with emotion. "We were very lucky that Isabel was there. She had experienced death in her family and knew that we needed her support in order to be able to see Jenny's body and say good-bye to her. She came into the bedroom with us. This act of kindness gave us the courage to see Jenny again, to caress her wrinkled hand, and to tell her that we would miss her."

◆　　◆　　◆

AND NOW, YOU. . .

Whether the death of your family member is expected or not, it almost always comes as a shock when it actually happens. Death brings your responsibilities for your relative to an end. Until now, you may not have been aware of how large a part caregiving has played in your life, and may be surprised by some of your feelings. You may feel sad, but also relieved that your relative is released from suffering, and that you are released from caregiving. On the other hand, you may feel numb, angry, or confused—all common and expected signs of grief. It may take some time for you to be ready to begin a new phase of life without your relative.

Well-meaning friends and family may also say things that seem insensitive or that hurt your feelings even though their intention is to be helpful and to comfort you. People are often very awkward around someone whose relative has just died. Their comments may be an expression of their belief that death is a blessing when someone is old or has been sick a long time. They may be trying to help you feel less sad about the death, or they may be trying to deal with their own sadness. But only you can know the meaning of the death and its impact on you. As you have learned from your career as a caregiver, it is best to let family and friends know what is and is not helpful to you.

Although each person grieves in his or her own way, many caregivers have found it helpful to join a bereavement group, which offers a safe place for the bereaved to express grief openly. You may, on the other hand, choose to work individually with a social worker or other mental health professional, or with a pastoral counselor. The Alzheimer's Association, hospices, and other community social agencies often offer groups or can direct you to the resources you need. (See Appendix.)

Keep in mind that in time you will gradually feel better and be able to bring renewed energy and interest to your life. In many cases it may be necessary to make new friends and explore new interests. This process can be both exciting and frightening.

Healing does not progress at a steady pace. Try to accept the inevitable setbacks, and take heart from your accomplishments. You will grow stronger by facing and dealing with new and difficult situations. It is one of the ways in which caregiving rewards the caregiver who has given so much and felt so much pain.

APPENDIX

DEFINITION OF TERMS
COMMONLY USED ON PRESCRIPTIONS

Abbreviation	Meaning
ac	before meals
bid	twice a day
hs	at bedtime
od	right eye
os	left eye
po	by mouth
pc	after meals
prn	as needed
qd	every day
qid	four times a day
tid	three times a day
q3h	every three hours
q8h	every eight hours
q12h	every twelve hours

DESCRIPTION OF HOSPITAL AND
SUPPORT PERSONNEL

Attending Physicians

Physicians who have completed all their training and can admit patients to the hospitals with which they are affiliated. They supervise the work of fellows, residents, interns, medical students, and physician assistants, and make all final medical decisions.

Residents

Physicians who have graduated from medical school, completed an internship, and are undergoing specialist training (i.e., general internal medicine or surgery). They will be involved in much of the day-to-day care of a patient, take medical and family history, complete physical examinations, order tests, write prescriptions, and administer any complicated procedures and treatments.

Interns

Interns have graduated from medical school and are completing their first year of post-graduate training. Like residents, they do physical examinations and history-taking interviews with the patient, and are responsible for ordering tests, tracking lab results, and charting detailed progress notes about the patient.

Physician Assistants

Physician assistants are trained in accredited programs to provide some of the same services as physicians. Working under the supervision of physicians, they can conduct physical examinations, diagnose and treat illnesses, order tests, assist in surgical procedures, and, in some states, prescribe medication.

Nurse Practitioners

Nurse practitioners have a master's degree in nursing and may have a specialization in a particular area of primary care. They can perform physical examinations, treat mild chronic conditions, and, in some states, write prescriptions under the supervision of a physician.

Nurse Managers (Head Nurses)

Nurse managers maintain supervision over all nursing activities on a unit, coordinate the duties of the nursing staff, and manage any difficult situations.

Registered Nurses (RNs)

Registered nurses perform a wide range of nursing duties, such as planning, assessment, and evaluation within the area of nursing responsibility. These include administering medications, narcotics, and IV fluids; changing dressings; counseling patients about procedures and treatments; and monitoring patient status.

Licensed Practical Nurses (LPNs)
LPNs perform duties such as taking temperature and blood pressure, changing dressings, and administering medications.

Nurse Attendants (Nurse's Aides)
Nurse attendants take care of a patient's non-medical needs, such as bathing and dressing, or helping a patient in and out of bed.

OTHER SUPPORT PROFESSIONALS

Chaplains
Most hospitals have chaplains representing several different faiths. They lead religious services, and offer counseling and support to patients and families.

Neurologists
Neurologists are medical doctors specializing in the diagnoses and treatment of disorders of the brain, spinal cord, and nervous system. They can diagnose AD and follow the neurological changes in the patient throughout the disease.

Nutritionists
Nutritionists counsel patients about nutrition and maintaining specialized diets while in the hospital and after hospitalization. They may specialize in areas such as diabetic or geriatric nutrition.

Occupational Therapists
Occupational therapists help recovering patients regain their ability to perform daily activities at home, work, and in the community.

Patient Representatives
Patient representatives explain patients' rights and responsibilities to patients and their families and resolve conflicts between patients and staff. They also explain how to use and fill out documents such as health care proxies, DNR orders, and living wills; and help to meet special needs, such as locating translators.

Physical Therapists
Physical therapists help recovering patients regain physical strength and mobility after injury, surgery, or prolonged illness. They may specialize in a particular aspect of therapy; i.e., orthopedics or neurology.

Psychiatrists
Physicians who specialize in preventing and treating mental disorders, and emotional and behavioral problems. They are often involved in the diagnoses of dementia and can recommend suitable medications and strategies for responding to its symptoms.

Psychologists
Psychologist study brain/behavior processes from a scientific viewpoint and apply this knowledge to help people understand, explain and change behavior and improve their ability to function as individuals and in groups.

Recreational Therapists
Recreational therapists use music, art, games, and other forms of leisure to stimulate a patient's physical and mental abilities.

Social Workers
Social workers offer patient and family counseling for difficult medical situations, coordinate discharge plans based on medical needs, and provide resource referral. They may also lead support groups, seminars, and educational programs for caregivers and patients.

Unit Clerks
Unit clerks are responsible for all administrative tasks on a given unit. They can provide information about which staff is assigned to a given patient or when a patient is scheduled for a test or procedure.

PROFILE OF A PERSON
WITH MEMORY IMPAIRMENT

This profile describes the special needs of a person with memory impairment. Its purpose is to help someone who does not know this person to understand how to take care of him or her. The profile describes how memory impairment affects the way this person behaves, the areas in which she/he needs help, and how to calm and comfort him or her. It also includes a list of current medications and allergies. It can be used at home, in the hospital or physician's office, and anywhere else special care and knowledge of this person are required.

Date form completed _____
                                                                    Mo/Da/Yr

Profile of _____ Date of Birth _____
                      First name   *Last name*   *Mo/Da/Yr*

Social Security #_____ Medicare # _____

Medicaid # _____ Other Medical Insurance _____

1. Primary contact _____
                                        First name   *Last name*

Telephone numbers *(home)* _____ *(work)* _____

Other contact numbers _____
                                        (Specify: Cell, Voice Mail, Beeper, etc.)

Relationship to the person with memory impairment

_____ Husband _____ Wife _____ Son _____Daughter _____Son-in-law

_____ Daughter-in-law _____Brother _____Sister _____Partner

Other (specify)_____

2. The person with memory impairment lives . . .

_____ With primary caregiver   _____ With another family member

_____ Alone at home   _____ In a nursing home

_____ With primary caregiver   _____ With another family member
          and paid caregiver   and paid caregiver

_____ At home with   _____ In an assisted-living
          paid caregiver   facility

_____ Other (specify)_____

3. Additional contacts

(1) _____ Relationship _____
       First name   *Last name*

Telephone number *(home)* _____ *(work)* _____ *other)* _____
                                             Specify: Cell, Voice Mail, Beeper, etc.)

(2) _____ Relationship _____
       First name   *Last name*

Telephone number *(home)* _____ *(work)* _____ *other)* _____
                                             Specify: Cell, Voice Mail, Beeper, etc.)

4. Person preparing this profile *(if not primary, contact)*

_____ Relationship _____
      First name   *Last name*

Telephone number *(home)* _____ *(work)* _____ *other)* _____
                                             Specify: Cell, Voice Mail, Beeper, etc.

5. Name of physician _____
                           First name   *Last name*

Address_____ Telephone Number_____

Hospital affiliation_____

6. Hospital to which the person with memory impairment should be taken in an emergency

_____

7. Information that will help people care for the person with memory impairment

Does this person speak and understand English?   *Yes*   *No*   *Don't Know*

If not, what language(s) does the he or she speak? _____

Does this person . . .	*Always*	*Sometimes*	*Never*	*Don't Know*
understand where he or she is?				
answer questions accurately?				
follow instructions?				
remember what he or she is told?				
tell others what he or she needs?				
tell others when he or she is in pain?				
use the telephone without help?				

Does he or she . . .	Always	Sometimes	Never	Don't Know
normally use a hearing aid?				
use eyeglasses?				
have dentures?				
Does this person normally need help feeding him or herself?				
If yes, does he or she need . . .				
food cut in pieces?				
to be helped to eat?				
to be fed by someone else?				
Does he or she need help with toileting?				
If so, does this person . . .				
indicate that he or she needs to go to the bathroom?				
need help finding the bathroom?				
need supervision while in the bathroom?				
need help with incontinence products?				
Is this person incontinent of urine?				
incontinent of feces?				
Does he or she need help . . .				
with personal hygiene (bathing, shampooing, brushing teeth, etc.)?				
with dressing?				
getting out of bed?				
Can he or she normally walk without a cane, walker, or person?				
If not, does this person . . .				
walk alone using a walker?				
walk alone using a cane?				
walk only with someone assisting?				
normally use a wheelchair?				

Does this person . . .	Always	Sometimes	Never	Don't Know
have good balance when standing and walking?				
fall out of bed?				

Does this person . . .	Always	Sometimes	Never	Don't Know
lose personal possessions such as glasses, etc.?				
get confused by new people?				
get confused in new places?				
get anxious or frightened if left alone?				
wander or pace?				
have angry outbursts or yell?				
get agitated or upset in the late afternoon?				
stay awake at night?				
become physically aggressive (biting, grabbing, spitting)?				
act in sexually inappropriate ways?				
have hallucinations, delusions, or paranoia?				
often get depressed, sad, or withdrawn?				

What helps calm this person when he or she becomes upset?	Always	Sometimes	Never	Don't Know
playing soothing music				
increasing the lights				
dimming the lights				
taking a walk				
offering food				
turning the television on				
turning the television off				
being with someone familiar				
being left alone				

Other things that help (specify) _____

_____

_____

8. **What medical conditions does this person have?**

_____

_____

_____

9. **What medications does this person take?**
(Be sure to include prescription and nonprescription drugs, vitamins, nutritional and herb supplements.)

Name of Medication	Dose	When Given	Name of Medication	Dose	When Given

10. **Is this person allergic to any medicines?**　　　_Yes　No　Don't Know_
If yes, which ones _____

_____

11. **Is this person allergic to any foods?**　　　_Yes　No　Don't Know_
If yes, which ones _____

_____

12. **Does this person need a special diet or**　　　_Yes　No　Don't Know_
consistency of food?
If yes, please explain _____

_____

13. **Is he or she enrolled in the Safe Return Program?** _Yes　No　Don't Know_
(If a Safe Return member gets lost, call 1-800-572-1122.)

14. **Has the person with memory impairment**　　　_Yes　No　Don't Know_
completed advance directives?
If so, where can they be found? _____

15. Personal history of person with memory impairment

What kind of work does (or did) this person do? _____

_____

What are (or were) his or her interests or hobbies?_____

_____

Is there anything else that is important to know about this person, such as special needs or plans?_____

_____

GUIDE TO RESOURCES

ORGANIZATIONS FOR PEOPLE WITH ALZHEIMER'S DISEASE AND THEIR FAMILIES

Alzheimer's Association
National Headquarters
225 North Michigan Avenue
Suite 1000
Chicago, IL 60601-7633
1-800-272-3900
www.alz.org

Referrals to local resources for caregivers and people with AD, such as support groups, educational information, and seminars. It also maintains the nationwide Safe Return Program, which helps families find people with Alzheimer's disease. Contact your local chapter to enroll your relative.

Alzheimer's Disease Education & Referral Center (ADEAR Center)
PO Box 8250
Silver Spring, MD, 20907-8250
1-800-438-4380
www.alzheimers.org

Educational materials on diagnosis and treatment of AD; patient care and caregiver supports; and education, training, and research related to AD. The staff will respond to telephone and written requests, and make referrals to national and state resources.

Alzheimer's Disease Centers (ADC's)
1-800-438-4380
www.alzheimers.org (Choose "Links to Other Federal Resources")

Information about federally funded centers that provide comprehensive evaluation for AD, treatment, and services—in addition to psychosocial research and clinical trials of new medications.

Clinical Trials Information
www.ClinialTrials.gov

This web site was developed by the National Institutes of Health to provide general information about clinical trials, and lists trials currently available for Alzheimer's disease and other conditions.

HEALTH INSURANCE AND BENEFITS INFORMATION

Medicare
1-800-MEDICARE (1-800-633-4227)
www.medicare.gov

Centers for Medicare & Medicaid Services (CMS)
(Previously, The Health Care Financing Administration, HCFA)
7500 Security Boulevard
Baltimore, MD 21244-1850
1-410-786-3000
www.cms.hhs.gov

Information for the public about Medicare and Medicaid programs.

Social Security Administration
1-800-772-1213
www.ssa.gov

People who are deaf or hard of hearing may call the toll-free "TTY" number, 1-800-325-0778, between 7 A.M. and 7 P.M. on business days.

ORGANIZATIONS THAT PROVIDE HEALTH CARE INFORMATION
AND ASSISTANCE TO THE ELDERLY

Resource Directory for Older People
National Institute on Aging
Public Information Office
Building 31, Room 5C27
31 Center Drive, MSC 2292
Bethesda, MD 20892-2292
1-800-222-2225
Available through the Administration on Aging web site at: *www.aoa.dhhs.gov*

Information about long-term care planning, nutrition and fitness (including meals on wheels programs), health promotion, etc.

The Eldercare Locator
1-800-677-1116
www.eldercare.gov

A nationwide directory assistance service designed to help older persons and caregivers locate local support resources.

American Association of Retired Persons (AARP)
601 E Street, NW
Washington, DC 20049
1-800-424-3410
www.aarp.org

Provides general information about health care, health insurance options, caregiving, etc.

National Association of Professional Geriatric Care Managers
1604 N. Country Club Road
Tucson, AZ 85716-3102
1-520-881-8008
www.caremanager.org

An organization of private practitioners (generally social workers and nurses), who develop and implement care plans for older people and their families. A Consumer Directory is available for $15 from the national office.

National Association for Continence (NAFC)
PO Box 1019
Charleston, SC 29402-1019
1-800-BLADDER or 1-800-252-3337
www.nafc.org

Resources for people with bladder and bowel control problems and their families.

American Academy of Family Physicians (AAFP)
11400 Tomahawk Creek Parkway
Leawood, KS 66211-2672
1-800-274-2237
www.aafp.org

Education of patients and the public in all health-related matters.

American Geriatrics Society
The Empire State Building
350 Fifth Avenue, Suite 801
New York, NY 10118
1-212-308-1414
Fax: 1-212-832-8646
Membership questions and information: 1-800-247-4779
www.americangeriatrics.org

Shapes attitudes, policies, and practices regarding health care for older people.

National Hospice and Palliative Care Organization
1700 Diagonal Road
Suite 625
Alexandria, VA 22314
1-800-658-8898
www.nhpco.org

Helps locate hospice services and runs a toll free hospice referral line.

National Association for Home Care
228 7th Street, SE
Washington, DC 20003
1-202-547-7424
www.nahc.org

Available through the Administration on Aging web site at: *www.aoa.dhhs.gov*
Helps locate accredited home care aide services and hospice information by area.

FEDERAL AND STATE AGENCIES THAT GOVERN HEALTH CARE IN THE US AND PROVIDE HEALTH-RELATED SERVICES TO THE GENERAL PUBLIC

The U.S. Department of Health and Human Services
200 Independence Avenue, SW
Washington, DC 20201
1-877-696-6775
www.hhs.gov

The principal federal agency that governs health care in the United States, providing over 300 health care programs such as Medicare, Medicaid, nutrition programs like Meals on Wheels, support services, and health care research. The Department of Health and Human Services web site gives an overview of all its agencies and links to agency web sites. Below is a listing of some HHS agencies that may be helpful in providing care for your family member.

Administration on Aging
330 Independence Avenue, SW
Washington, DC 20201
General Information: 1-202-619-0724
Statistical and Gerontology Information: 1-202-619-7501
www.aoa.dhhs.gov

Contact information for state offices of the aging, the eldercare locator, long-term care ombudsman programs; resources for locating birth certificates, property deeds, and other records; resources for financial and legal planning and other topics of interest to the elderly.

National Institutes of Health
9000 Rockville Road
Bethesda, MD 20892
1-301-496-4000
www.nih.gov

Information about current health care research, clinical trials for various diseases and conditions, and research centers that provide evaluations for Alzheimer's and other diseases.

National Institute on Aging
Building 31, Room 5C27
31 Center Drive, MSC 2292
Bethesda, MD 20892
1-301-496-1752
www.nia.nih.gov

One of the 25 institutes and centers of the National Institutes of Health that focuses on the study of aging. It is the primary federal agency involved in Alzheimer's disease research and provides information about the topic to the public.

The Centers for Disease Control and Prevention (CDC)
1600 Clifton Rd.
Atlanta, GA 30333
1-800-311-3435
www.cdc.gov/health/seniors.htm

General health care information for the elderly.

Agency for Healthcare Research and Quality
2101 E. Jefferson St., Suite 501
Rockville, MD 20852
1-301-594-1364
www.ahrq.gov/clinic

Information about health care research that is designed to help patients and families make educated decisions about care.

ADDITIONAL RESOURCES

The 36-Hour Day: A Family Guide to Caring for Persons with Alzheimer's Disease, Related Dementing Illnesses and Memory Loss in Later Life, Nancy L. Mace and Peter V. Rabins, Johns Hopkins University Press, 1991.

One of the most respected books about the care of a person with Alzheimer's disease.

Video Respite
From: Innovative Caregiving Resources
P.O. Box 17809
Salt Lake City, Utah 84117-0809
1-800-249-5600
www.videorespite.com

A series of videos featuring music, light movement, and interactive entertainment specially designed for Alzheimer's patients. Individual videos and other products can be purchased from Innovative Caregiving Resources.

Geri Hall, PhD, ARNP, FAAN
University of Iowa School of Nursing

Geri Hall is a well-known nurse practitioner who offers consultation on coping with Alzheimer's disease to patients and family members. She can be reached by email: geri-hall@uiowa.edu.

ACKNOWLEDGMENTS

This book is the best way we can imagine of showing our appreciation and admiration for the family caregivers who gave freely of their time to share their personal experiences in the struggle to maintain the health of their relative with Alzheimer's disease. In celebrating their efforts, we trust that they will be pleased with ours. We hope that what we have done here will help ensure that the needs of those diagnosed with AD are met with dignity, and their health care is provided in accordance with the highest possible standards.

This work could not have been accomplished without the involvement and encouragement of the following foundations and individuals:

The Grotta Foundation for Senior Care, under the guidance of Susan Friedman, has believed in the value of this project from the moment it was proposed and, along with the FJC, provided financial and emotional support throughout. Their generosity supplemented the resources of the NIA-funded NYU Alzheimer's Disease Center.

A special thanks is due to the staff of the Silberstein Aging and Dementia Research Center. Family counselors Emma Shulman (CSW), Gertrude Steinberg (MA), Alicia Pierzchala (CSW), Helene Bergman (ACSW), and Migdalia Torres (CSW) made enormous contributions. Drs. Barry Reisberg, Steven Ferris, Alan Kluger, James Golomb, Emile Franssen, and Isabel Monteiro, whose work is in the vanguard of AD research, patiently answered all our questions.

We are also grateful to those who reviewed and offered helpful comments on the manuscript during its development. Members of the hospital staff at NYU provided the perspective of professionals who work within the health care system, and ensured that the recommendations and suggestions in the book would be realistic and workable. They include: Jackie Bier (RN, MA, CS), Director of Nursing in Medicine; Gail DiStefano (RN, MA), Director of Critical Care, Nursing Department; Veronica Flynn (RN), Nurse Manager, and Maureen Schechner (RN), Senior Nurse Clinician, Emergency Department. Marilyn Lopez (MA, RN), Geriatric Nurse Practitioner, Tisch Hospital, whose compassion for her elderly patients was always inspiring to us, came up with timely resource material whenever we needed it. Dr. Martin Finkelstein, Professor of Geriatric Medicine, with his reviews and incisive suggestions, called our attention to critical issues. Esther Chachkes (DSW), Director of the Departments of Social Work and Therapeutic Recreation, and Eileen Zenker (MSW) made themselves available for consultation on discharge planning. Sandra Burke, Director of Patient Representative Department, responded with wit and wisdom to each request for information on advance directives and other ethical issues.

The concepts and research on the medical care of an Alzheimer's patient developed by Geri Hall (Phd, ARPN, FAAN), Associate Director for Outreach, University of Iowa Center on Aging, informed the work throughout. Fred Brand, former Director of Program and Services of the New Jersey Alzheimer's Association, Lois Hull, Director of Special Projects of MDNJ, and members of the caregiver support group at NYU also reviewed the manuscript with intelligence and insight; as did Della Frazier Rios, caregiver and Director of Training and Education at the New York Alzheimer's Association. Staff members of the NYU Medical Center and UMDNJ, and family caregivers participated in focus groups that highlighted and clarified the problems faced in their common goal—meeting the needs of dementia patients in the hospital.

Phoebe Hoss created the structure and many of the basic concepts of this book; Barbara Ravage, manuscript editor, made invaluable contributions to the content as well; and Martin Smith added the finishing touches. We also wish to thank Janet Reichert for invaluable help in preparing the manuscript for publication.

Thank you all.

INDEX

A

AARP (American Association of Retired Persons), 187
activities, 44–45
activities of daily living (ADLs), 158
acute, 5
Administration on Aging, 189
adult day care programs, 18, 45, 47
advance directives, 10, 50–53, 108, 168–69
Agency for Healthcare Research and Quality, 190
aggressive behavior, 130, 132–33
agitation, 130–32
aides, 119, 177
alcohol use, 20
Alzheimer's Association, 18, 185
Alzheimer's disease (AD)
  See also dementia
  cause of, 4
  as cause of dementia, 3
  communicating diagnosis of, 41–43
  defined, 3–4

medical problems caused by, 9–11
medications for, 34
stages of, 5–9, 11–12
symptoms of, 3–4
Alzheimer's Disease Centers (ADCs), 186
Alzheimer's Disease Education & Referral Center, 185
ambulances, 72–74
American Academy of Family Physicians, 188
American Association of Retired Persons (AARP), 187
American Geriatrics Society, 188
anxiety, 40
artificial nutrition and hydration, 52
assisted housing, 163–64, 166
attending physicians, 176
autopsies, 171

B

bed sores, 142
behavior
  aggressive, 130, 132–33
  agitated, 130–32

dealing with disturbing, 46–47
restrictions, 20–21
strategies for managing problem, 130–35
behavioral, 5
bereavement period, 172–73
board-and-care residences, 163–164

C

cardiopulmonary resuscitation (CPR), 52
caregiver
  emotional well-being of, 101–5
  feelings of, 104–5
  role of, during doctor's visits, 25–26
  role of, during hospitalization, 96–100, 136–42
  role of, in emergency room, 78–80
  stage of dementia and, 11–12
  support for, during hospitalization, 100–5
catheters, 79, 142

Centers for Disease Control and Prevention, 190
Centers for Medicare & Medicaid Services (CMS), 186
chaplains, 177
chemical restraint, 116
chronic, 5
cigarettes, 20
clinical drug trials, 35–37
Clinical Trials Information, 186
cognitive, 5
comfort care, 52
communication
    with Alzheimer's patient, 137–38
    with hospital staff, 123–24
    between patient and hospital staff, 137–38
competence, 107
congregate housing, 163–64
continuum of care retirement communities (CCRC), 163
contracture, 142
crisis kit, 62–63
crisis planning, 61–68
    See also emergencies
    arranging for care to/at hospital, 63–65
    crisis kit for, 62–63
    hospital information for, 65–67
    insurance issues, 67
custodial care, 158

D
daily routine, 40
death
    See also end-of-life issues
    advance directives concerning, 10, 50–53, 108, 168–69
    after, 170–73
    autopsy after, 171
    decisions to make before, 167–68
decision making
    about end-of-life issues, 108–11, 167–68
    advance directives and, 10, 50–53, 108, 168–69

help with, 110–11
during hospitalization, 106–13
including patient in, 49–51
medical, 48–53, 106–13
delirium, 5, 9–10
delusions, 7, 46–47
dementia
    See also Alzheimer's disease
    cause of, 3–4
    defined, 5
    mild, 6–7
    moderate, 7–8
    moderately severe, 8
    role of caregiver and, 11–12
    very severe, 9
dental care, 19–20
Department of Health and Human Services, 189
depression
    defined, 40
    treatment for, 45–46
diapers, 79
diet, maintaining healthy, 20–21
discharge plans, 143–47
disorientation, 130
DNI (do not intubate), 109
DNR (do not resuscitate), 109–10
doctors
    choosing, 15–18
    following recommendations of, 85–86
    questions for, before hospitalization, 65, 86–87
    second opinions from, 112–13
    specialists, 19
    visits to, 22–28
        caregiver's role during, 25–26
        making easier, 24–25
        noncooperation during, 26–28
        preparing for, 23–24
drugs. See medications

E
eating disorders, 10
Eldercare Locator, The, 187

emergencies
    See also crisis planning
    ambulance transportation for, 72–74
    identifying, 69–71
    preparing for, 71
emergency rooms
    care provided in, 75–76
    discharge from, 80–81
    hospital admissions from, 80–82
    procedures of, 76–78
    role of caregiver in, 78–80
    toileting procedures in, 79
emotional well-being
    of caregiver, 101–5
    improving, 44–45
    maintaining, 39–40
    sharing news and, 43–44
    telling about Alzheimer's diagnosis and, 41–43
    treating depression, 45–46
empty day syndrome, 44
EMTs (emergency medical technicians), 72
end-of-life issues
    See also death
    advance directives for, 10, 50–53, 108, 168–69
    decision making and, 108–11, 167–68
    palliative care, 169–70
environment modifications, 39
exercise, 11, 142

F
feeding tubes, 10
food preparation, 21

G
geriatric chair, 116
geriatric social workers, 18, 178
geriatricians, 15–16
group homes, 163
guardianship, 107

H
Hall, Geri, 191
hallucinations, 7, 46–47
health care

See also doctors; medical treatment
dental care, 19–20
importance of regular, 13–15
outside of doctor's office, 18
from specialists, 19
health care proxy, 52
health problems
delirium, 9–10
eating disorders, 10
incontinence, 10
movement problems, 10–11
importance of treating, 14–15
hired help, 117–20
home care
additional, 157–58
after hospitalization, 146–47, 151–59
medical equipment for, 156–57
preparing for, 152–53
services for, 154–56
when it becomes too difficult for, 159
home care agencies, 154–55
home health aides, 155, 158
hospice care, 169–70
hospital rooms
arranging, 129
making comfortable, 128–35
hospital staff
alerting, about dementia, 97–98
building relationship with, 122
communicating with, 123–24
communication between patient and, 137–38
expectations from, 122–23
helping them understand Alzheimer's patient, 124–25
roles of, 125–26
types of, 176–78
working with, 121–27
hospitalization
accompanying person for, 63–65

advance planning for, 61–68
crisis kit, 62–63
insurance companies and, 67
questions about hospital, 66–67
questions for doctor, 65, 85–87
respite services, 67
alternatives to, 84
caregiver's role during, 96–100, 136–42
deciding on, 85–86
decision making during, 106–13
difficulties of, 92–93
effect of, 91–95
emergency, 69–74
encouraging cooperation during, 138–40
hiring help for, 117–20
immobility during, 142
living arrangements after, 146–47, 161–66
managing behavior problems during, 130–35
nursing home placement after, 162
preparing for, 87–88
returning home after, 146–47, 151–59
care needed, 157–59
preparing for, 152–53
services for, 154–56
short-term care after, 161–62
special needs during, 95, 115–20
stage of dementia and, 93–94
supervision during, 114–20, 117
support for patient during, 81–82
support for caregiver during, 101–5
hospitals
discharge from, 143–47
emergency rooms, 75–82
getting comfortable in, 102
social support in, 103
transferring between, 71
housing arrangements. *See* living arrangements

I
immobility, problems caused by, 142
incontinence, 10
insurance coverage
for home care, 145–46, 154, 157–58
requirements for, 67
interns, 176
invasive procedures, 10

L
licensed practical nurses (LPNs), 119, 177
life-sustaining treatment, 52
living arrangements
See also home care
adjusting to new, 165–66
after hospitalization, 146–47, 161–66
choosing, 164–65
nursing homes, 162
subacute-care facilities, 161
types of, 163–64
living will, 51–52

M
medical equipment, 156–57
medical problems. *See* health problems
medical treatment
decision making about, 48–53, 106–13
advance directives for, 10, 50–53, 108, 168–69
help with, 53
including patient in, 49–51
encouraging cooperation with, 138–40
second opinions about, 112–13
Medicare, 186
medications
for Alzheimer's disease, 34
clinical trials of, 35–37
helping with, 31–34
importance of taking required, 29
pharmacists and, 30
problems with, 140–41

strategies for taking, 32–33
understanding prescriptions for, 30, 175
memory loss, 3–4
mental competence, 107
mental health care, 38–47
movement problems, 10–11

N
National Association for Continence, 188
National Association for Home Care, 188
National Association of Professional Geriatric Care Managers, 187
National Hospice and Palliative Care Organization, 188
National Institute on Aging, 189
National Institutes of Health, 189
neurological, 5
neurologists, 177
nurse managers, 176
nurse practitioners, 18, 176
nurse's aides, 119, 177
nursing homes, 160, 162, 166
nursing supervision, 155
nutritionists, 177

O
occupational therapists, 156, 177

P
paid companions, 119
palliative care, 169–70
paranoia, 7
patient representatives, 119, 177

permanent vegetative state, 52
personality changes, 8
pharmacists, 30
physical restraint, 116, 117
physical therapists, 156, 178
physician assistants, 176
physicians. *See* doctors
power of attorney, 51, 52
prescriptions, 30, 175
Profile of the Person with Memory Impairment
defined, 58–59
form for, 179–84
using, 59–60
progressive, 5
psychiatric symptoms, 46–47
psychiatrists, 178
psychologists, 178

R
range-of-motion exercises, 142
recreational drug use, 20
recreational therapists, 178
registered nurses (RNs), 119, 176–77
rehabilitation therapy, 155–56
residential care facilities, 160
residents, 176
Resource Directory for Older People, 187
resources, 47, 185–91
respite services, 47, 67
restraint
chemical, 116
physical, 116–117
retirement housing, 163
routine, daily, 40

S
safety issues, 21

self
taking caring of, 101–5
sheltered housing, 163
skilled nursing care, 158
smoking, 20
Social Security Information, 186
social service organizations, 45, 47
social support, 103
social workers, 18, 178
speech therapists, 156
subacute-care facilities, 160–161
sundowning, 131
support groups, 18, 46–47, 103
support system, caregiver, 100
surrogate decision maker, 52
symptoms, 5
of Alzheimer's disease, 3–4
medications to treat, 34
progression of, 5–9
psychiatric, 46–47

T
television viewing, 44–45
therapists, 155–56, 177–78
transportation, by ambulance, 72–74

U
unit clerks, 178

V
Video Respite, 190
violent behavior, 92–93, 133
visiting nurse, 155
Visiting Nurse Service, 18